'MUMMY, WHY HAVE I GOT DOWN'S SYNDROME?'

When Elizabeth Joy was two years old, Caroline wrote a moving account of the pain and joy of having a Down's baby. The book *Elizabeth Joy* was warmly received and won much praise. Over 20,000 copies were sold.

Lizzie is now nine. In this new book Caroline Philps brings Lizzie's story up-to-date, and looks at her life today. How does Lizzie relate to her younger brother and sister? How do they respond to her? How does having a Down's child affect family life? What about school? Lizzie's father is a clergyman: how does Lizzie react to church? What about holidays? How does it feel to be Lizzie's Mum? What has it meant to be Lizzie's Dad? What is life like, now that Lizzie is growing up?

Once again Caroline Philps crystallizes the joys and dilemmas facing parents with Down's children. Her story is one of hope, and the book she has written is a valuable source of information.

Caroline and her husband Mark, with their three children—Lizzie, Nick and Susie—live in the industrial West Midlands of England. Caroline is a teacher as well as a writer: she is currently undertaking research into the language development of Down's children.

For Mark, Nick, Susie and Lizzie,
who is as excited about this book as
if she had written it herself

'Mummy, why have I got Down's Syndrome?'

Caroline Philps

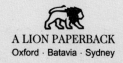

A LION PAPERBACK
Oxford · Batavia · Sydney

Copyright © 1991 Caroline Philps

Published by
Lion Publishing plc
Sandy Lane West, Oxford, England
ISBN 0 7459 1921 9
Albatross Books Pty Ltd
PO Box 320, Sutherland, NSW 2232, Australia
ISBN 0 7324 0471 1

First edition 1991

Acknowledgment
The author acknowledges with special thanks the work of
Mrs Sue Gillette 'who has patiently deciphered my writing and
typed most of the book for me'.

British Library Cataloguing in Publication Data
Philps, Caroline
    Mummy, why have I got Down's Syndrome?
    1. Down's Syndrome children. Philps, Caroline
    I. Title
    362.3
    ISBN 0 7459 1921 9

Printed and bound in Great Britain
by Cox and Wyman Ltd, Reading

CONTENTS

A bird with clipped wings
cannot fly

But you shall fly
dearest child of God;
you shall fly

Yet you shall be different
bitter sweet
blessing and burden

In their aloneness
may your family
be close together

In their reaching
may you not doubt their motives:
always loving

And in their nurturing
may their protection
not be a bitter boundary

Fly, Elizabeth Joy, fly!
little bird with clipped wings

This poem was specially written
for Lizzie by Jane Grayshon

Introduction

It is difficult to describe any person adequately. It is even harder to describe someone who is so much an essential part of our lives as Lizzie is. This book is not neutral, it can't be. It is also selective, it has to be. But I hope it is positive. Because Lizzie has enriched our lives in a unique way.

Growth is often painful. Growth into parenthood is, I believe, for many parents, sometimes a painful process. It is part of growing up. For us, there was also the pain of coming to grips with what having a handicapped child might mean.

But it is not through gritted teeth, but often with amazement and laughter that we continue to get to know our daughter. She has helped us see the world through new eyes and our other children—who are equally special to us—are part of that world.

So this book is for anyone interested in children. But perhaps it is especially for the many parents who share our own particular experience, in the hope that it may bring encouragement as they face the future.

I hope that, as you read this book, you will meet Lizzie through its pages. I hope too that you will find in it reflections of yourself and of the God who made and loves us all.

CAROLINE PHILPS

PART ONE

THE FIRST EIGHT YEARS

'*True love is an act of will that often transcends ephemeral feelings of love.*'

Scott Peck, *The Road Less Travelled*

1
Birth

I shut the front door quietly, so as not to wake the children, and walked towards the car. It was just beginning to get dark, and I felt a twinge of excitement as I unlocked the car door.

Settling myself comfortably, I pushed the tape into the machine and allowed myself a moment to revel in the luxury of going somewhere on my own. Then I nosed the car out of the drive and onto the busy road.

But apprehension intruded as I drove through the streets of Victorian houses, past the factories, on the route to the hospital.

Where was the maternity block?

With relief I saw the signs, found the entrance hall and at last stood by the lift.

By now my heart was thumping and I felt slightly sick. As the lift rose up to the second floor, I hugged the red photograph album closer and tried to rationalize my feelings.

I felt I was on some kind of mission. Yet I knew I could not take responsibility for the family I was visiting.

I approached the nurses' station. 'The pediatrician asked me to visit,' I said. I followed the sister to a side ward and realized, as I approached the door, that the personal chat I'd hoped to have with the mother would not be possible. Several relatives surrounded the bed and I felt an intruder. I wished I had been able to come in the daytime.

I smiled gently at a friendly older woman who must have been the new grandmother. I saw a beautiful, although very pale, young woman sitting up in bed. Her young husband looked distracted and did not seem to welcome me.

I tried to explain why I had come and the husband said I could have a few minutes to talk. He asked the rest of the family to wait outside.

Feeling even more uncomfortable, I hesitantly placed a small parcel on the bed. 'I brought this for the baby,' I said. The mother looked surprised but seemed pleased.

I wanted to put myself in their shoes, but time heals and changes us. It was hard to remember what the pain and the shock felt like. Maybe they would think it had been all right for me.

The trouble was that I did not feel sad any more. Cross sometimes, but not sad. Mostly I felt joyful as I thought of the funny bundle of mischief asleep in her bunk. So how could I help this couple, except by showing that we can survive these things and still be human.

I started to talk. 'I have a Down's child too,' I began. I wondered if they would dislike the label as much as I had? 'She is eight years old now. I have some photographs. I know you must be feeling very shocked at the moment.' I tried to control my voice, not to be too enthusiastic, to take account of their grief.

The doctor had told me they were planning to leave the baby in the hospital. That worried me. The idea of total abandonment. Yet I wanted to understand.

Unbelief was still written on the father's face. Why had this happened to them? They were only twenty-three. He was too young for the responsibility.

Remaining in hospital was painful for the mother. She intended to go home next day. She couldn't stand being surrounded by these four walls any more. I understood that feeling. They felt so hurt, they had to return to the safety of their home. But distanced from the birth of their daughter it might be easier to reject her.

'Would you like to see her?' the father was saying. I felt

11

momentarily hopeful; I sensed a note of pride in his voice. We went towards the lift. The sick feeling returned.

This was so like the journey I had made from post natal ward to the special baby-care unit on the days following Elizabeth's birth. Every hospital lift stirred this kind of emotion in me. I had been hurting, then, just like this man. He confided his sense of despair as the lift descended. I tried to say that it did get better. That the responsibility would not be too great. But his grief would not let him hear or believe. It was too soon.

The lights were bright in the tiny room in Special Care. The red lino reflected the glare. I peered into the small incubator, and the tiny baby looked red too. Her thick black hair stood up from her head. 'Would you like to hold her?' She was placed in my arms. My heart was pounding again and my stomach churned as I gently held her.

For a moment this was not someone else's baby—she was mine, and my heart ached for her...

Saturday 11 April (1981)
I cried a lot last night. A nurse brought me in some tea and said, 'You'll be all right. You've got faith, haven't you?' Why are my personal beliefs suddenly everyone else's property? How does she know it will be so easy? 'They don't know who brings them up anyway,' she went on. Was this meant to be consoling? I'm so glad I spent two university vacations working at a hospital for mentally-handicapped children; and glad about the little girl I met last summer—far better than reading a description in a book. They *do* know who cares for them and who loves them.

Was it only last night the pediatrician asked to see my husband? The nurse told me when I first went to see my new daughter at 5 p.m. I thought there must be something wrong and I looked down at the tiny person in my arms: an expression, or was it the shape of her face, reminded me of something. And then I knew. 'She's a mongol, isn't she?' I said to the nurse. 'They don't know yet,' she replied. But *I*

12

knew. I bravely said that I was a Christian and God must have a good purpose in giving her to us. The nurse praised my attitude. But I said to my daughter, 'You'll be the brainiest mongol out,' and I tried hard not to cry.

Mark came as soon as I'd managed to telephone him—I hated telling him over the phone—I felt guilty. He'd just been telling our family and friends that we had a daughter. Now he would have to phone again. I felt I'd failed him. I hadn't managed to have a normal baby, like the other mothers in the hospital. I was relieved to discover that Mark had spent half an hour with her when I was being stitched up. He hadn't noticed anything wrong then and just thought she was a very sweet little baby. I sensed that he loved her, despite everything. But I tried to be brave for him.

The pediatrician arrived and told us it was possible that we had a Down's baby. I hated the label. It made it hard to think of her as a person. He was sending blood samples for tests and we would know within a week. He was caring, yet he talked so easily about something that had just completely changed our lives.

When I awoke this morning, very early, I thought for a second that it was all a terrible dream. Then the sickening thud at the pit of my stomach told me otherwise. I spent the day in utter desperation longing to see my daughter. I asked several nurses when I could go down and couldn't believe it when they said I'd have to wait until after their tea-break. When eventually I was escorted towards the special baby-care unit the excitement and tension mounted.

I'd only held her for half an hour in the first twenty-four hours of her life. Would I love her? Would the gap of time when I hadn't seen her put a barrier between us? Could I accept her? Why did I have to fight the feeling of revulsion and alienation when I thought that her body wasn't made in quite the same way as ours?

I pushed open the swing doors. And there she was—such a tiny creature. I hated the stockinette cap and mittens taped over her hands, the aertex nightie that swamped her. It made

13

her more alien. I wanted to cuddle her, and the hat kept falling off or into her eyes. She was wrapped up tightly in a sheet and given to me to hold. I felt very angry when I heard she had cried for half an hour when they'd been too busy to feed her. I wanted to be here with her. I sat in a chair in a room full of incubators and held her close and talked to her.

A nurse came up later and told me I would tire her out. How could love tire someone out? Someone who needs all the love there is, I thought fiercely. I want to make up for not being allowed to be with her. She is my little daughter, not government property.

She reminds me of my great-grandmother. The moment she was born I saw her face—was it the slightly shrivelled appearance of new babies or the little, straight, closed mouth over no teeth? Now as I looked down at her I fought back the tears—maybe they were relief. I knew I loved her. It was heaven to hold her close to me. I hated having to put her back in her cot but she was very tiny and I was told she needed to rest.

Sunday 12 April
I was allowed to move down to the special baby-care unit today. I couldn't believe that I could have my daughter with me all the time. I just lay on the bed and listened to her breathing...it was so amazing to think that she belonged to me. She had such tiny hands and face.

I read my Bible for the first time since she was born. Psalms 61 and 62 were the reading for the day, and one verse jumped out at me from the page: 'You have heard my promises, O God, and you have given me what belongs to those who honour you.'

That was how I was meant to understand our little daughter, as a gift, a special gift. We had thought we would call a daughter Sarah, but somehow it didn't fit. As I thought, I felt that we should call her Elizabeth, Elizabeth Joy. Elizabeth because this means 'gift or promise of God', and Joy because I knew we should be confident that she would bring us much joy. It was an act of faith at this moment but we could be sure God would honour that faith in him and in our daughter.

I went on to read, 'God is my strong protection and shelter, his love is constant.' I felt I knew the truth of this verse in the hospital now. I felt very vulnerable, and yet I knew that underneath me and around me were the strong arms of God. He would keep me holding on to him. I couldn't pray and yet I sensed I was with God all the time and that somehow it didn't matter.

Wednesday 15 April

I have felt today as if I've become the butt between the conflicting ideas of the two nurses in charge of the ward. They do not seem to agree about how Elizabeth should be fed, how many times I should try to breast-feed and how many bottle or tube-feeds she should have. I can't cope with it. The pressure to get her to suck seems so great, it feels as if she will never be able to come home. Yet at midnight tonight I tried to feed her myself and she tried so hard to suck the nipple. She started crying because she was so frustrated that she couldn't succeed. Or at least that was how it seemed to me. I was thrilled that she exhibited such normal emotions.

Thursday 16 April—Maundy Thursday

Today I came to the end of myself. I couldn't cope any more. Perhaps intellectually I'd accepted Elizabeth's birth in the first few days. It hit my heart today.

After lunch the drugs that I'd been given to help my womb contract properly began to act rather powerfully. I was unprepared for this and panicked. I was waiting on tenterhooks, too, because I felt sure I'd overheard the doctor talking about whether I could go home with Elizabeth. I couldn't bear the suspense. I thought I was going to pass out. 'I can't stand it any more, any more,' I yelled at the nurse who brought me some pain-killers. I felt very angry that I hadn't been warned the drugs would make me feel awful and that all

15

I needed was to take something with them. Why hadn't anyone told me?

It was amazing to find my feelings so closely mirrored in the Bible reading for today, from Psalm 39: '...my sufferings only grew worse, and I was overcome with anxiety. The more I thought, the more troubled I became; I could not keep from asking: Lord, how long will I live?' When I was told that I could go home with Elizabeth I just couldn't believe it. I felt like a prisoner being set free...or even as if I'd come back from death. This really is Easter, not just in the time of year but in the events in my life.

As I pulled the huge babygrow onto Elizabeth's tiny floppy limbs I dared to begin to think that this really was my little girl; I was free to look after her in the way I chose now. I needn't live in fear that I wasn't obeying the rules of this nurse or the other, and I could even breast-feed her when I wanted to, without being told that I would tire her out. Perhaps my life was beginning again.

2
A Kind of Death

We brought Elizabeth home. Tears of relief streamed down my face as I carried the tiny bundle into the large dim house and shakily climbed the stairs to place her in the newly-bought cradle, a special gift from her Granny. It was bliss to put the new sheets and covers over her instead of the hospital ones. When Elizabeth started to breast-feed, after my one attempt at mixing the formula milk, I was very relieved.

The first days at home had a dream-like quality. The new freedom I experienced after feeling caught between the different regimes of the special baby-care ward and the post-natal ward was like being released from prison. I loved just walking down the road to the shops. I felt almost as if I'd returned from the dead. Life seemed so precious and time such a gift.

But I had been hurt and battered by the hospital experience and it was some weeks before the pain began to surface and I could admit the hurt I had felt at the words of some of the nursing staff, and the events of the first few days.

It was some weeks too before I could verbalize the loss and the sadness that I felt. All kinds of things acted as triggers: a television programme of children playing made me weep for the child we had lost who might never play on a swing. A visit from a friend with a baby the same age made me jealous of the firm strong baby, already more active than my own. And there was the day Elizabeth's medical card came, with Miss E. Philps on the envelope. The name seemed like a symbol of eternal spinsterhood: perhaps she would never marry.

Yet alongside the sadness was the novelty and delight in this tiny person who had entered our lives: her first smiles, and her lovely big blue eyes, her tiny star-fish hands reaching out for me as she fed; that tiny person for whom even first-size baby clothes were too big.

And there was excitement as we began to realize that Lizzie responded to us, she was learning and beginning to play. She was a human being after all.

The tensions and conflicts were too big for us.

The literature from the Down's Syndrome Association gave us plenty of ideas for early stimulation and exercises. 'This child is a challenge,' said the baby exercise sheet. There were books of medical hints. The stumbling-block was the label 'Down's'. We'd first heard it used (instead of mongol) late on the day Elizabeth was born. I remembered a desk and a doctor, apologetically, yet also in matter-of-fact tones, stating that it was likely this baby was 'Down's'. The label stuck in my throat, but we got used to it.

The problem was that the label, and lists of physical features, made me feel I had given birth to an alien creature, not our daughter. It took me months of rediscovery to realize that Lizzie looked like us, she had more of our genes—not fewer—than our other children would have. She was not like all other Down's children because none of them was really like any other. She was a little girl with a genetic mix-up. She had a problem, but she was herself.

As I faced the anxiety of the first serious illness, battled with the too-early mornings, with times when I was bored at home, with loneliness, I began to realize that at least some of my feelings were those common to all new mothers in the first few months. My times of depression were not solely because our child was different.

And the joy and fun of discovering a new person who responded and reacted—at a slower pace but still growing and moving forward—that too was the same as for other parents.

But I couldn't marry these two opposing streams of

thought. There was a kind of protective wall that I'd created round myself at the beginning and only slowly could I let the light in. It was easy at home where Lizzie was the centre of attention, to feel happy. This was our norm: feeding her, dressing her, playing and talking to her, hearing her baby noises.

It was only as we left the security of our own life and moved to touch other people's that we noticed the difference, and that was when it all hurt so much. She wasn't as firm and active as other children. Her face did look different. Her clothes didn't fit as well. Her face was rather round.

Our first holiday with Elizabeth was an oasis, perhaps because we were sheltered from the reality of the outside world by the strong, thick stone walls of that much-loved Cornish house, by the branches edged with lichen and the soft Cornish air. This was the place where Mark grew up. There was a familiarity, a continuity with our past. We could be our old selves without the new life contradicting that. Lizzie was a special granddaughter. There was no one else to tell us it was not so.

The future frightened me because of its uncertainty. The hospital had said no predictions could be made about Lizzie's ability. A group of handicapped adults disembarking from a coach onto a beach on holiday transfixed me. I made myself watch them. Would Lizzie become like that? What was the worst we could expect? Could we be prepared?

Yet there was hope. The future of these folk had been determined before the 1971 Education Act, which had laid down that handicapped children should be educated and not just looked after, let alone the 1981 Act which said they should be integrated into mainstream education. They were born before the Portage Project and pre-school education, vitamin therapy, wide-spread use of antibiotics and the Down's Syndrome Association. Average IQ was said to have risen from twenty-eight at the beginning of the twentieth century to about sixty by the 1970s. Life expectancy was now near normal. We had much to be grateful for.

Yet a conflict existed in my mind. I couldn't simply accept that Lizzie was just a little girl who had a few permanent problems. In those first weeks as I pushed her out in the pram I was often stopped by people, well-wishers, women out shopping. They saw the little person, propped up to look out and to play with her toys strung across the pram, and said 'What a sweet little baby.' I always said, 'Yes, she is...but she has Down's Syndrome.' I felt compelled to say it, but why this confession? Did I feel guilty or did I need their sympathy and concern? They didn't always know what to do with the information but I somehow felt better for saying it.

When some of the elderly women at church asked me if she was a 'good' baby, I felt like screaming inside as I said, 'Yes.' It would have seemed more normal to me if I'd said, 'No, she screams all the time.' I'd read about how 'good' Down's babies were—placid, even unresponsive. I went home and weeded the garden, tears running down my face. I stabbed at the soil furiously with the fork. I could not understand the anger under the surface.

I was very defensive—a sign of the problems I had in coming to terms with what was our loss. We had lost a normal healthy intelligent child. We were not sure who we'd been given instead.

Yet that was not the whole picture. There was a determination. If our child was damaged, we would do all we could to help her have a good chance in life. We would read and devour all the books and research papers we felt were relevant. I would plan exercises for her and enjoy the momentary joy of buying her something I felt would help her. The red toy-box in the corner of the sitting-room burgeoned.

Perhaps, too, there was pride. If we couldn't have a bright and alert normal child, we'd try very hard to have a bright and alert Down's child.

There may have been nothing wrong in that; but there was a pressure. I couldn't just relax and let her learn. I felt that if I worked hard enough with Lizzie I could change things for her. I had to learn that she was not just a pliable puppet, and we were not God.

To my mind there is only one thing that makes sense of all these contradictions. I believe there is someone who in fact takes these things, even our sometimes misdirected and mismotivated desires to change things and brings good out of it all. In his book, *The Problem of Pain*, C. S. Lewis said, 'God whispers to us in our pleasures, speaks in our conscience but shouts in our pains: it is his megaphone to rouse a deaf world.'

Since the day of Lizzie's arrival I had known a sense of God's planning of events; I had known his support. Even at the time when I felt most painfully that my world had fallen apart, God was there—a rock-like reality that perhaps I had never needed to experience so much before.

Lizzie's birth at Easter underlined for us the paradox of life coming through death. We felt our own hope kindled in the new life we were just beginning, with a new set of values as a base-line.

God's way was not to be successful as we think of success. His way is to take the poorest, most insignificant, weakest person and make something wonderful and special of them. Jesus was born in a refugee situation, with an animal feeding-trough as a crib, in meagre Bethlehem—not in a teaching hospital in Jerusalem. He died a criminal's death. Yet through him God chose to redeem humankind, removing the barriers of sin and disobedience to reunite us to himself.

God did not choose the wise, he chose the weak of this world through whom to display his glory.

We were beginning to learn this new reality in our own lives. Our vicar's sermon on the first Easter Sunday after Lizzie's birth was based on a verse from the New Testament: 'At all times we carry in our mortal bodies the death of Jesus, so that his life may be seen in our bodies...death is at work in us.'

.hen I first heard it I felt it was a strange choice for Easter
.day. But then I began to understand the relevance of it.
Easter was about death as well as new life: the one producing
the other.

It seemed so relevant to us at this time. We had to give up
our old dreams for our children. We had to let go of our way—
a kind of death—and let God have his way. After all, that is
what being a Christian really means.

One of the ways that God helped us to live our new life was
to provide some practical help through the Portage Project.
'Portage' was first developed in Wisconsin, in the USA. It is a
pre-school developmental stimulation programme based on
daily activities that are taught by the parent. A Portage
teacher is assigned to each family and visits on a weekly
basis. This weekly visit is crucial to the success of the project
because it provides support for the family as well as expert
help in suggesting suitable activities to be taught to the child.

Chris, a nursery-nurse friend of ours, had felt she should
go on a Portage training course. She had trained while I was
still expecting Lizzie. When Elizabeth was born, Chris was
available to come and help us. This made me feel that God
was at work, providing what we needed even before we knew.

In the early days, having a daily structured programme of
activities and exercises to do with Lizzie and a weekly visit
from Chris gave me encouragement. I had a structure to my
day, I had goals to achieve. I had someone concerned and
realistic about Elizabeth's progress, available to come and see
me. It did much to alleviate my feelings of depression. The
Portage visit was a highlight of the week.

We would lie on the brown carpet in the sitting-room, near
the nursery fireguard that enclosed the meagre gas fire whose
heat seemed barely to reach the high moulded ceiling. With
toys scattered around us, Chris and I would check that Lizzie
could still put the brick into the shape-sorting box, the man
into a hole, find the toy under the cloth. When it came to
crawling, we made slow progress—lures of toys would not

22

work too well. We put sweets out for Lizzie to crawl towards and I felt like a dog trainer. Later—much later—we would stand, one in each room, across the hall, telling her to 'take the dolly to Chris, please', 'give this to Mummy.' There would be shrieks of delight and some giggles as the penny dropped and she carried out the command.

It was exciting when Lizzie showed she really could do something. Early progress was often quite fast. But there were times of seeming stagnation when I got worried. Probably we'd chosen something Lizzie wasn't interested in, or ready for, but it wasn't always easy to know. It was fun when it worked. We often laughed, Chris and I.

Life was not just full of Portage. There was swimming at the local hydrotherapy pool. There were walks on the nearest patch of wood and common, parish activities, the youth group who were great fans of Lizzie, shopping, toddler club, distant friends who sometimes called in. A Portage conference for home visitors and parents came later in Lizzie's first year.

There was plenty to keep me busy and yet there was an inner loneliness, a feeling of not really belonging and of being different that coloured many meetings and many events.

There were family parties, Lizzie's baptism, Christmas, the day Mark was ordained as a priest. Yet all were tinged with a kind of sadness, and a sense of transience. We did not permanently belong to this community despite their warmth and love. We would move on one day soon. Even motherhood had not bound me to the other mothers. There was a difference I could never dismiss.

Occasionally my sense of loneliness plummetted into self-pity and introspection; then I tried to fill my days with activity. But often the tears were real grief—I flung myself onto the sofa, pressed my face into the fabric and sobbed after watching a television play about a Down's baby who was abandoned in hospital after birth. The agony of that little baby rejected and alone was just too much.

Lizzie continued to grow and develop. She sat up, propped

23

in her high-chair, later supported by a foam wedge, then at seven months on her own. She was quite podgy at that age, with a round face, but as she became more active, moving around in her round baby-walker or bouncing from the door-frame in her harness, she became slimmer and her face grew heart-shaped. Her lovely big eyes and sweet grin made her very lovable.

Yet subconsciously I was very aware of her appearance, feeling she did not match up to other people's babies. Other people's babies seemed to look nice in whatever they wore but only certain things flattered Lizzie. Why was that? Was I further from accepting Lizzie, exactly as she was, than I believed at the time?

There were moments of great delight: when Elizabeth was only six weeks old she made her bell fall off the end of her tray. She repeated this several times. It seemed a huge break-through. She had realized that she could move objects by herself.

At Christmas, when Lizzie was eight months, she learnt how to play her xylophone sitting on the floor in the sitting-room in Cornwall. Gradually she became more confident about walking. It was not until the following autumn, when she was about nineteen months that, after walking up and down beaches on holiday with cot sheets under her armpits, she walked on her own. My delight when she walked twenty-two steps around the sitting-room knew no bounds!

Lizzie was her own person from the beginning. She was not a placid child. She got angry if her lunch did not arrive quickly. She invented her own bouncing games—she wanted to be caught if she bounced off the settee and she laughed every time we caught her. She loved shredding tissues or crawling off with her nappy in her hand at bedtime when I needed to put it on. (The latter made me laugh, but shredded tissues have never amused me, and it took Lizzie years to stop enjoying that one.) She was a determined, independent character.

Some of the Portage activities were definitely unpopular

and she would not comply. We spent what seemed like months teaching her to release things. Only if the game was interesting would she join in. I felt fed up, it seemed as if she was making no progress. I encouraged myself by studying various developmental checklists and logging Lizzie's progress each month. I could then look back and reassure myself that she had moved on. I feared that she would not go on progressing, that she would sit still, that she would never grow up.

Maybe it was defensiveness that made me so upset when an acquaintance came round with her small boy. She said 'He can say fifty words now. What is Lizzie doing?' I don't know how I didn't scream at her. I cried afterwards at what seemed to me to be self-centred self-confidence. But doubtless it was only well-meaning tactlessness. I was still too sensitive to cope with it. Deep down I was afraid Lizzie would never speak, let alone say fifty words.

I did not have the confidence, then, to let go of the Portage activities Lizzie did not like and allow her to choose something she was interested in. I did not have the confidence I now have that babies will naturally learn and discover. Although Lizzie needed planned activities to lead her in the right direction, she too had that in-built desire to learn and investigate, even if it wasn't what I thought should be top priority. She might, for instance, investigate yoghurt drawings on her food tray, or the results of pulling her friends' hair!

I still struggled with a feeling of worry if Lizzie wasn't doing her Portage sheets or something 'constructive'. And this caused a good deal of tension with Mark. From the start he had not shared my then almost obsessive need to 'teach' Elizabeth things. The literature I had read just after she was born had so impressed me with the necessity of early stimulation that I came to believe her life depended on it.

Perhaps Mark was more philosophical. Being less of an activist, not driven by the urge to make the most of every minute, Mark found it easy to talk and play with Lizzie without evaluating each occasion as a 'learning experience'. He often complained about my zealousness. At the time, I felt he did not care about Lizzie learning or support me in what I was trying to do. It made me sad. Now I see it was partly to do with our different reactions to Lizzie's birth. When she arrived, I asked what I could do about it; Mark got on with accepting her as she was. Which he did.

Mark was not around when other mothers came with their children or I went to the clinic. He did not make the endless subconscious comparisons. Maybe that made it easier for him to accept; maybe I was less secure.

The conflict over Portage remained all through the time that Lizzie followed the programme. Our holidays were often times when the conflict emerged into open acknowledgment. For it was then that I felt relaxed and unpressured and wanted to spend more time helping Lizzie. It was then that Mark hoped for 'time-off' from routines.

I felt unsupported. Mark felt irritated. I felt as if I had to carry the burden for Lizzie's development. Yet Mark was a loving, caring and involved father. There were tears and arguments but neither of us could change the way we felt.

But, subtly, changes were coming. I began to see Elizabeth more and more as our daughter who happened to have some problems, rather than seeing her as a Down's child who happened to be our daughter. I began to realize that it didn't matter if sometimes she seemed typically 'Down'sish'.

For instance, one day when she was about twenty-one months, I wrote in my diary: 'This morning, after breakfast, Elizabeth sat on the floor by the door into the kitchen and banged her head against it several times. Then she rocked backwards and forwards for a few minutes. It didn't last long and I suppose she may have been experimenting with parts of her body. It is not obsessive and she doesn't often do it. But today I laughed. "This is typical behaviour of a handicapped child," I thought to myself, "and I don't care—I really don't. I love Elizabeth...I love Elizabeth exactly as she is."'

During the months that Elizabeth was learning to walk and to develop more independence, I was also moving forward into a new phase of my life. I was expecting our second child.

I found the early months of the pregnancy worrying. I refused an amniocentisis (a test involving sampling the amniotic fluid to see if the baby had spinabifida or Down's Syndrome) and the blood tests that preceded that, but I had mixed reactions from the hospital. The nurse involved understood my refusal to have an abortion and therefore refusal to have the blood tests: I did not want anxiety throughout the pregnancy if the blood test showed a problem. The gynaecologist was less helpful. I had had a traumatic experience when I was about twenty-three weeks pregnant and thought I was going to miscarry. I was taken to the same hospital department where Elizabeth had been born. It was a false alarm but my confidence was badly shaken.

I was comforted by Chris, our Portage teacher, who showed me a Bible verse that she felt was meant for us. God said, 'I will protect you as you travel and bring you to the place which I have prepared.' Remarkably, on the day I had probably conceived this baby a healing service was held at church. A Sri Lankan Christian spoke, and then prayed for Elizabeth and myself, amongst many others. I had had a real sense of God's presence in that service and now, looking back, I wondered if God was saying, 'This child is part of my healing for Elizabeth and for you.'

Gradually my confidence returned. As the baby grew larger and moved and kicked I dared to look forward to the birth.

Although I had been devastated by the emergency visit to hospital I had learnt a lot. It was not wrong to want a normal baby, it was the most natural thing in the world. But it was better to hang on to God and his promises to me, because he was trustworthy, rather than pin all my hopes on the baby itself. Peace came in those last few months and also a sense of excitement.

The move that we needed at the end of Mark's first curacy was offered us: a second curacy in an area only ten miles away. It was a pleasant area of suburban London, bounded by forest. There was a park and a lake at the bottom of the garden of the house we would live in.

We could move before I was due to have the baby. That meant I could have the 'domino system'. I would see my doctor and midwife for regular check-ups before the birth, and then the baby would be born in the general practice unit of the hospital—my midwife and doctor attending. I was booked in with a midwife who was a member of our new church, and the Christian doctor she worked for. If all went well, there would be only a six-hour stay in hospital.

This all seemed such a wonderful answer to my unexpressed prayer. I felt I could not endure returning to the hospital where I had had Lizzie. I saw God's hand, too, in the healing that would come from a good birth experience with our second child. God was at the centre of our everyday life, healing the hurt and also leading us forward. At the same time, the sense of loss was not just something that was to be healed—and that would be the end of it. The loss, the feeling of brokenness which we experienced in Lizzie's birth had a positive side, in that it enabled us to share with others who had also experienced pain.

In the last few months before we left Mark's first curacy I visited someone of whom we were very fond, although we didn't know her very well. She was dying of cancer. Although our pain had been small in comparison with hers, having Lizzie gave me courage to go and see her.

In those last few months before we moved, Lizzie was becoming a little girl rather than a baby. She would sit at a small table in the sitting-room doing jigsaws, or playing with a tiny sand tray, scribbling or chalking. For her second birthday she was given a slide by her Granny. At her party she stood at the top in her tights, skirt and jumper, about to go down. A photograph captured that moment for me: Elizabeth with a grin on her face, a little girl now, ready to move on. Her red cheeks were shiny, because of the colds she often had when teething.

The psychologist who assessed Elizabeth before we moved told us that her general development was close to average but the main area of delay, as we knew, was her spoken language. This was at about an eighteen-month level. Potty training and feeding were also behind. But her level of play was good and she was willing to learn.

I felt then that the struggles we had had to persevere with the Portage work had been worthwhile. We had been able to help build a foundation for the future and maybe we could relax a little as she began to learn more by herself.

The educational psychologist said that Elizabeth would learn most through normal playgroups and nursery school. At some point later on she would need some form of special education, but we must beware of specializing too early. She would possibly benefit too from the early years of a normal infant school, as long as she was given some extra help. We left his office with relief and joy. It was an affirmation that my belief in her was not a distorted mother's view but a true picture.

At the time, my relief was too fragile a thing to enable me to consider how other families might have felt as they left a similar interview with perhaps a less hopeful prognosis.

We moved house. Looking forward to new beginnings, we suddenly grew nostalgic about the place we had left behind, the place where Lizzie had come and changed us. There would never be another place quite so full of contradictory memories, both of pain and of joy.

During Lizzie's first two years, we had come to know ourselves better. We had come to recognize the downward spiral of self-pity and learnt to set our minds against it, to trust God, to be grateful. This kind of mental discipline was something Mark had recorded in his diary just before Elizabeth was born and in the days after:

9 April

'Endure hardship as discipline' (Hebrews 12:7). I suppose the real secret lies in our attitudes. We can treat life as full of the inexplicable and chafe against it, or we can accept anything that is hard to understand or cope with as a form of God's discipline. That way everything is capable of being turned to good account.

11 April

Funny I should have read that verse two days ago—before what happened yesterday. 'Everything is capable of being turned to good account,' I wrote. If this child is a mongol, may God turn that to really good account, that his name may be glorified...

13 April

Yesterday was Sunday, with these words in the epistle, 'the foolishness of God is wiser than men; and the weakness of God is stronger than men'. Surely this all ties up with the strange ('foolish') idea that this little girl is a trust from God. We are tempted to say, 'It's all a mistake,' or, more theologically, 'It's part of the fallenness of nature.' But we feel that she was meant, and we cannot wrap our minds around that, because the foolishness of God is wiser than we are. All suffering, supremely the suffering of Christ on the cross, is part of the foolishness of God. It doesn't make intellectual, philosophical sense, but at a deeper level its wisdom is palpable. And so, to suffer is to be close to God, because in some way we are able to see, without being able to explain, what he is doing in the world...

Our memories form complex patterns. Our feelings about the places we live in are coloured by the pain and joy we experience there, and not just by the bricks and mortar or the trees or lack of them or the people that we know. I remember our first family home in a kind of kaleidoscope of dark and light of feelings, indelibly impressed on my mind and heart.

30

The furnace where gold is tried and tested is not remembered afterwards for its heat but for the work done in creating something beautiful. Perhaps for us this place had a furnace-like quality. It was a place we didn't want to return to, not because we didn't care about the people, but because it meant returning to painful memories. And yet it was a place neither of us would have missed for the world.

3

A New Beginning

In June that year, 1983, I wrote, 'The summer has come at last and the garden is full of roses. A summer's day has ended with a clear blue sky and tinges of pink and orange between the rooftops.

'In a brown wicker cradle lies a little boy. He is just drifting off to sleep. His name is Nicholas. In the next room sleeps a little girl who is not quite sure if the advent of this small creature is good or bad. She likes to stroke his head and hands, to hold him, but the endless feeds and attention he receives cause her to feel insecure and sad.

'But to us Nicholas has brought a sense of completeness. The two years of a kind of isolation from the world of normality have ended. We are parents as others are parents, without the pain and sense of loss.

'Nicholas is healthy and contented. He arrived a week early, quickly and easily. He is someone who will one day be able to understand that he has a special sister.

'A few hours after he was born a sudden wave of sadness washed over me, as I realized that Elizabeth could have been like Nicholas. Whole, normal, with the right number of chromosomes. But I pushed away the tears that flowed easily in the aftermath of giving birth. We had been given Elizabeth as a special gift—a kind of bonus child. We can and will rejoice in her. Her smile, perhaps the more appealing because it emphasizes her Down's features, will always bring us joy. She is our special child and Nicholas will one day be grateful that he has known her.'

Nicholas was a hungry baby. I found it hard to keep up with the feeds. I would drive recklessly back from Lizzie's playgroup, Nick screaming in the carrycot strapped on the back seat, screaming for all the ten-minute drive. He had to be fed in many places, in the farmyard corner at the Cotswold Wildlife Park, in the car, at supper, on the beach, in the night—many times in the night. But it was summer, a beautiful hot summer which didn't end until the beginning of September when we went on holiday. Then the gales began and our first holiday with two children was at times a kind of nightmare. Nick had a temperature. We visited the beach with a full quota of anoraks and wellies. Lizzie didn't have much sense of adventure at the age of two and the waves looked fierce and noisy.

But it had been a beautiful summer. I could push our brown pram all around the lake and the woodland at the bottom of our road. The sun through the trees made beautiful patterns and textures on the rutted ground.

Lizzie was reluctant at first to sit on the child-seat on top of the pram. It was exposed and open. But there were lovely sunny afternoons when we walked across the park and up the hill to the clinic. I would be exhausted at the end of the return trip, but seeing the ducks and swans on the lake and feeling a sense of freedom within me more than compensated.

There were walks in the other direction too. Up the road, to the shops on the green. By the golf course with the lightning-charred tree trunk pointing a long finger to the sky. Past the hall where the playgroup was held, then past our own church, the white and blue wooden building where Mark led the services each Sunday. Up to the shops on the green and the duck ponds and the old buildings.

I did feel free. Free at last from the emptiness inside me. Here, in our new home, everything felt different. The beauty of the trees alone was almost enough.

There were people I could go to coffee with, where I could be me, just a mum with two children, not 'the curate's wife'. But perhaps the personal affirmation I felt was more to do with the tiny baby in the pram and the sense of healing and joy he brought than I realized at the time.

It was not boring to have to juggle the time-tables of two children and a husband needing to be fed—I enjoyed the challenge. I had to fit Lizzie's Portage activities into times when Nick was happy or asleep. I had to fit shopping into times just after his feed when I knew I had an hour or so clear of crying and tetchiness. I had to fit in Lizzie's visits to a local playgroup, where they welcomed handicapped and normal children together. There were also her visits to our local Children's Centre, where she received ear, eye and speech checks. There was a playgroup there once a week while the mums discussed the latest Open University course 'The First Years of Life' or some other relevant topic. I was busy. And it was lovely.

Then Nick got a high temperature. The temperature didn't go down and he screamed if moved. I phoned the doctor. By the time he arrived Nick was shaking. The doctor was worried and drove us straight to the hospital for admission. Meningitis, he wondered?

I couldn't bear to think I might lose this baby. I delighted in him. He was beautiful. But the fear lasted until the test results were through. Not meningitis but a week in hospital while Nick had a series of antibiotic injections. I slept on a fold-up bed in the same room, so that I could feed him, and after a couple of days he began to smile again and to move about in his cot. He would be all right.

Lizzie was at home with Granny. I went home when I could, to have a bath, to read Lizzie a story...

On our wedding anniversary Nick was discharged and I pushed the children up to the Family Service at the parish church on the green with my mother. Freedom again. It tasted wonderful.

Nick grew so quickly. It wasn't long before he sat on the floor playing with his toys while I worked with picture matching or some other game with Lizzie.

Lizzie seemed to have accepted the advent of a new

member of the family. I'd bought her a baby-sized doll so that she had her own baby to feed. It was realistic enough to be mistaken for a real baby from a distance and periodically frightened us by its face-down poses on the carpet. Later it lost all its hair, was renamed 'hairless baby' by another member of the family, and lost its power to confuse.

But Lizzie wanted to pick Nick up too and carry him around. I could never leave them alone together. As Nick was awake for longer periods it was difficult constantly to watch them and cook the supper or go to the loo. I hated tea-times, especially if Mark was late back from visiting people or from a meeting, and couldn't hold a child or keep Lizzie occupied while I cooked a meal. I didn't want the contents of the kitchen cupboards on the stone floor several times a day. I often felt frustrated and angry.

Putting out the washing was an operation that filled me with dread. Our garden was reached by a long flight of very steep steps, because it lay about ten feet below the house. How was I to get Lizzie, Nick and the washing safely down, without Lizzie immediately following me back up the steps once she was in the garden. If I left her, she cried and might fall down the steps. If I left Nick upstairs in the house he cried. We put up gates and barriers at top and bottom. Then I had to climb over them with large baskets of washing.

As the leaves began to turn to brown and the days became colder Lizzie continued her two mornings at the private playgroup. The helpers tried to do some of her Portage activities. They were kind. But it was a big hall and Lizzie was shy. When Nick was eight months I wrote in my diary 'Lizzie hasn't spent more than two minutes at anything today except getting tissues out of the box and 'dusting' with them. She is teething. I get very frustrated.

'Nicholas is teething too, but also he is learning to put objects in containers (something Lizzie found extremely hard) and says 'mama' and 'dada'.

'Lizzie is saying some new words: 'owl' and 'door'. She can read 'chair' and 'door' from labels stuck on to these objects.

She can say about forty-five words now. She enjoys doing very simple jigsaws, although she finds the idea of matching parts of the pictures very difficult.'

Later my diary recorded something that preoccupied me almost continuously at this time. 'I am worried that I feel I love Nick more than Lizzie. I saw an old friend last week and she said she had felt the same every time she had had a new baby and it all evened out in the end.' I was somewhat comforted by this. But the feelings and the guilt connected with it continued. It was so easy to enjoy Nick and all he did; I agonized over the anger I felt towards Lizzie. Where was my determination to accept her as she was? I was disappointed when she played with tissues or undid a loo-roll or made a mess at a friend's house. Would she never grow up?

Language was our great preoccupation that year. All the Portage activities were based on encouraging Lizzie to speak. We had to be careful how they were organized as asking Lizzie to say a word had no result whatsoever.

Mollie White, a Portage teacher in Winchester, and Kathy East, had developed an elaboration of the language section of the Portage checklist. The Portage checklist itself was divided into five areas: socialization, motor skills, self-help, language and cognitive skills. Because the checklist covered 0–6 years, the language list in particular often left large gaps between skill levels and it was hard to bridge them.

Speech is the area needing most work for nearly all Down's children, so the new 'Wessex Revised Portage Language Checklist' helped to bridge those gaps as well as linking up other language-related skills from different areas of the Portage checklist. I found it helped me to see where Lizzie's language was developing and where we needed to concentrate on improving it.

Makaton was also something we tried to use at this time. This is simple sign language which is used in schools and in the home to help non-speaking children to communicate. The idea is that if a child is confident signing a word, this may help them to speak it. The adult who signs always speaks the

36

word too. Lizzie learnt the sign for 'biscuit'—a tap of the palm of the hand on the opposite elbow—very quickly. We learnt about a dozen of the Makaton signs, but gradually Lizzie's speech began to develop and I often forgot to use them.

Language development in Down's children was also being researched at Portsmouth Polytechnic by Sue Buckley. She discovered that by teaching young Down's children to read before they could fully speak, their language was improved. Down's children seem to find it easier to see something and to speak using the written word as a prompt, rather than to hear and copy orally.

I had found that Elizabeth loved books and pictures from a few months old, and we decided to follow Sue Buckley's ideas. We selected photographs of common objects. (Learning Development Aids produce a set of photographs that a psychologist, Bill Gilham, developed, based on the same ideas.) We then made name labels to put underneath. To begin with, Lizzie matched the name to the picture. Later she read the name alone, and later still she began to build sentences using the known cards.

Over a period of about three years I worked with Lizzie on this process and by the time she was five she was able to read simple sentences, even though she might not speak the sentences in her own conversation.

One Wednesday in February, I went up to the parish hall where a women's lunch was being held. The speaker's subject was trusting God and his promises. She had placed a promise out of the Bible on every seat in the hall and when we arrived we read ours. Lizzie's verse moved me with its relevance (despite the masculine sounding language): 'Blessed is the man who perseveres under trial, because when he has stood the test, he will receive the crown of life that God has promised those who love him' (James 1:12). There would be trials for Lizzie and she would have to persevere. Mine was from Psalm 16 verse 8: 'I have set the Lord always before me; because he is at my right hand, I shall not be shaken.' It was to prove more relevant than I could have foreseen at the time.

At the end of March, *Elizabeth Joy*, the book I had written covering the first two years of Elizabeth's life, was published amidst—for us—unexpected and unprepared-for publicity. I was excited and yet also fearful about the sharing of our own personal and private experience with so many unknown people.

The back page of *The Times* always carries a Bible verse. On publication day I could hardly believe my eyes—it was the verse God had shown me the day after Lizzie was born. The verse that made sense of it all: 'You have heard my promises, O God, and you have given me what belongs to those who honour you.' Here it was again, on publication day. I had been sure God had a purpose in my writing the book. This confirmed it.

Large black-and-white photos taken of Lizzie for publicity at this time show her proudly holding a copy of her book. When she was born, I had certainly never imagined that all this would follow.

In early May I took the children to Wolverhampton to stay with my sister for a few days. Taking two toddlers on a train was an endurance test I had no wish to repeat in a hurry, and Lizzie had cystitis for the first time while we were there, something she was to suffer from several times in the next few months.

Then, the day before Nick's first birthday, I was rushed into hospital with peritonitis. I was in hospital for ten never-ending days with complications following the operation.

I recovered quickly, all things considered, and in July we were able to borrow a cottage in Swanage for a few days for a beach holiday with the children and then to go across country to a Christian holiday based at a boarding school in Sussex.

After the holidays I wrote in my diary: 'I need to write about the difficult things we are experiencing with Lizzie at the moment. She seems very rebellious. She has her own ideas, and if we don't give in to these she has tantrums. She is very independent and I feel she is testing us out.

'Potty training has taken fifteen months and she is still wet three times a day and often does a pooh in her pants. I feel so fed up every time I see the tell-tale brown patch on her trousers or skirt, or the puddle on the floor. It was a nightmare on holiday in a large building to sort that out.

'When Lizzie gets bored she refuses to walk anywhere at all. It makes us feel we can't ever go on walks again. We love walking, even if it is just a short walk in some woods. Lizzie doesn't see the point of walks. Yet when we come back and she finds some toys or a slide to play on she'll have plenty of energy again.

'She scratches and hurts Nick and takes his toys. Maybe Nick will be damaged by all the aggression. What effect does it have on him? He screams loudly enough, but I don't enjoy that. Lizzie insists on undressing in public, in unsuitable places. It makes me feel ashamed of her—that I can't have trained her properly. It's my fault. Everything is out of control.

'Lizzie generally refuses to do Portage tasks. That causes tension and a feeling of failure too.'

I comforted myself with the memory that she played without too much fighting on the beach and that she ate well. But it was not enough to compensate for other memories.

On holiday in Sussex, we had to drive her around in the car in the evening to get Lizzie to sleep. I felt very resentful that despite babysitting arrangements which we never had at home, we couldn't enjoy the delicious candle-lit suppers arranged for the adults. One of us had to keep a meal for the other while Lizzie was lulled to sleep. Again I felt we had failed. We couldn't be like everyone else and enjoy ourselves.

Lizzie wakes up at 5.30 a.m. most mornings, so we feel constantly tired. On holiday, where breakfast was at 8 a.m. it seemed an interminable wait. (I would end up in the empty dining-room at 7 a.m. feeding her Weetabix and longing to go back to bed. But the early morning walks with her round the grounds that looked over the North Downs were some compensation.) Someone has to be on 'Lizzie duty,' as she cannot be allowed unsupervised anywhere at the moment. She is three and I feel very disheartened, specially when I see other children of the same age. I feel the toddler stage is going on a long time, it is wearing and she is testing us out. She screams all the time when I try to wash her hair and when I try to cut her nails. I have to be so physically firm with her that I'm sure I must hurt her just to hold her still. For a moment, sometimes, I even feel I *want* to hurt her for making life so difficult. Yet how terrible to admit that truth. I want to praise God for Elizabeth but it seems impossible when I feel so angry.'

In public I put on a brave face. I played it down because I felt that was what we should do. I shouldn't feel angry. It was wrong, wasn't it? I also felt Lizzie's uncontrollable behaviour must somehow be my fault. So perhaps I deserved it all, anyway.

On the holiday, I felt so desperate that I sought out one of the leaders. I asked if I could pray with her about my feelings towards Lizzie. Sitting uneasily in her room, I began, 'I'm worried because I feel I love Nick much more than Lizzie. I feel very guilty about it. I often feel very angry with Lizzie. I'm worse when I'm with her at home on my own. I'm better when other people are around.'

To my relief, Liz replied, 'I felt the same about my son, although he had no special problems.'

We prayed together and the sense of relief at verbalizing my tangled feelings supported me through the rest of the holiday. I realized that I needed to stop trying to be self-sufficient. I was encouraged too by Liz's words of admiration for my handling of Lizzie. I needed encouragement.

But everything got more difficult before it began to improve...

4
Nursery School

In the autumn Lizzie started at a nearby nursery school. She was three and had a morning place. I pushed Nick and Lizzie in the double buggy down the steep hill, cutting through the small piece of woodland which acted as an irresistible magnet to me. (The path was rutted but it had the benefit of going beneath a leaning tree trunk that became a bridge.) The footpath felt dangerously close to the lorries that thundered down the lane, but it was soon passed, and I humped the buggy over the curb, to cross by the traffic island to the long low buildings of the school. I followed in the wake of the other mothers and children and walked up the path to the nursery unit.

The glass doors were brightly painted with Miffy characters in bold black outlined simplicity, and the playground was full of climbing apparatus and interesting grass hummocks and paths.

Inside the large room were areas for wet and dry play, paint, dressing-up, a hairdresser's and a Wendy house. The book corner had tiny chairs and cushions and there were trays of materials for building models or threading, matching or sorting.

Two rooms led off the larger room and the children were divided into two groups: yellow and green. Each of these was broken down into small groups of children—everyone allocated their special day of the week when they wore a badge and had a special book to write in. That day they were monitors: the plums or oranges or strawberries. (It all depended on what the very hungry caterpillar had eaten on their day of the week, because names were based on the *The Very Hungry Caterpillar*—Eric Carle's marvellous picture storybook.)

It was a wonderful place, full of light, enthusiasm and life. There was always plenty to do and although Lizzie began in the sand and water areas and spent weeks experimenting there, she gradually began to move into the house corner and played more imaginatively. Conversation would take a long time to develop, and to begin with she was often an observer.

When I collected her after her first morning I was anxious to know how the teachers would feel about having their first Down's child. For weeks I felt obliged to ask rather worriedly if she'd been all right. For several days she came out clutching a plastic bag full of wet, or—worse—soiled pants. I would carry them to the car, a sense of failure marring my pleasure at feeling Lizzie had been somewhere where she would learn.

Gradually, as Lizzie became used to the routine, and as the nursery-nurse (who also happened to be her Sunday School teacher) worked out a routine for taking her to the toilet, the accidents became fewer. But it wasn't until the end of the school year that we were able to find the beginnings of a solution.

Miracles are part and parcel of the Christian faith. As a Christian I believe that God became man, that Jesus healed many people during his earthly life, that his death on the cross was followed by the miracle of the resurrection. During the Autumn, Mark attended a conference about the healing ministry of Jesus and how that could be part of the experience of today's church.

On the last evening I took Lizzie along to be prayed for. I was beginning to be aware of the difference it would make if Lizzie could tell us what she did at nursery, say how she felt. I longed for her to be able to speak properly. We felt excluded from many areas of her life, not because she didn't want to share them but because she couldn't. So I asked for prayer that her speech would develop and also for her chest to be stronger, because she often suffered from croup. As we went home we decided we should try to pray for Lizzie in this way regularly.

Our kitchen looked out through the branches of an enormous apple-tree, growing from broken crazy paving, ten feet below. As the trees lost their leaves and I could glimpse the grass of the park beyond our fence, and the thorny rose bushes bereft of colour in our rather unkempt garden, I would stand and stare while I washed up at the sink or stirred a pot on the stove.

I was often tired in those days, and somehow dissatisfied and frustrated. But there was fun too. I helped the children colour-match socks in the laundry pile (an idea from the Open University course I'd been studying) and then we put the things in the washing-machine. They both climbed into the empty washing-basket which was waiting for its load of wet clothes, and sat and ate the cheese biscuits that they had for mid-morning 'elevenses'. Their new boat caused plenty of giggles.

Dressing-up in old hats and scarves kept in the ancient picnic basket on the landing upstairs provoked squeals of delight too. Lizzie wore a red hat on top of a scarf and clutched a handbag, and Nick, in an old felt school hat with a straw basket at his side, was not to be outdone. The fact that they were often in their sleepsuits on the way from or to bed added to the fun. At least, so the photographs tell us.

They were often great friends and in many ways they were almost like twins. At Christmas Lizzie was three and Nick was nineteen months. Lizzie had begun to have a passion for Postman Pat. She loved watching the programme on television and hearing the stories. It was the first time she expressed a special enjoyment of something herself and I was so pleased to be able to buy her some Postman Pat toys for Christmas.

Everything was Postman Pat—from the bendy toy,

jigsaws and games, to the jumpers Granny sent from Cornwall with Pat, the van, and Jess the cat on the front.

It was fun to watch her delight on Christmas Day.

Our collection of games was increased after Christmas and we began to play simple colour-matching games together—'match the balloon' was one. On some good days Lizzie and Nick would both sit up at the white melamine table we had in the living-room and do jigsaws together, or use Play-Doh or do drawing. By January Lizzie was reading about twenty words from cards and using some Makaton signs. Cutting out and tracing were improving too. There was great competition between them and Nick's main word was 'mine', perhaps because Lizzie delighted in tormenting him, taking his toys and scratching his face whenever my back was turned.

Lizzie's jealousy was never verbalized, but it was frequently demonstrated, and I went through agony every time. An agony of frustration and anger that she had to be so spiteful, upset that Nick had to take the brunt of it, yet sometimes feeling Nick made such a fuss that he almost 'asked' for another attack.

I would put them in the double-buggy ready to go out to the shops or to school. I would leave them for a few seconds to fetch a bag or go to the loo, and I'd return to a screaming Nick, a scratched face and a triumphant Lizzie. What was I to do? I despaired.

I despaired about other things too. I wrote in my diary: 'I feel worried about Lizzie's short concentration span and her shouting and bad behaviour. I end up shouting at her and it colours the day. I feel a failure as a mother and I fear that Lizzie's bad behaviour is my fault. Yet Nick is much more reasonable, so perhaps it is to do with Down's Syndrome and not to do with me.'

During this particular year my own frustration and anger at repeated, and what seemed to me pointless, kinds of behaviour, began really to concern me. It caused a great deal of inner conflict as I felt the power of my anger and rage.

44

It was often sparked off by the inability of Nick and Lizzie to remain playing peacefully for more than one second after I left the room. It was also sparked off by the inevitable dirty pants at the most inconvenient moments.

It was always when we were about to go out, or were somewhere miles from a loo, and I hadn't got all the equipment, or we were late already. And there it would be, the tell-tale enlarging brown stains on Lizzie's trousers and the bulge I knew I had to sort out. My panic button was pressed...I often stamped furiously up the stairs, or—worse—up from the garden and then up the stairs, if the garden was the place where it had happened. I held too firmly to a struggling, crying Lizzie and left an inevitably crying Nick somewhere he didn't want to be left.

I stood Lizzie on the loo floor, and tried fruitlessly to remove her trousers without getting all the mess on her shoes. Failing to do that successfully, I then tried to remove the unwanted contents of the pants, and the pants themselves, without dropping everything on the floor. The ritual was accompanied by my shouting at Lizzie, or, if it was a really bad day, screaming at her or muttering swear words under my breath, about which I would spend the next few days feeling remorseful. My remorse would turn to depression as I viewed my inability to cope and be 'Christian' about it all.

There was, inevitably, a lot to clear up after one of these events. Lizzie would have to be bathed, and the floor and the clothes washed. If we were due out somewhere my panic and anger would rise as we became later and later. Nick would be screaming downstairs, or from the cot where he had been parked for safety. If it happened while we were out, I felt embarrassed and inefficient.

Now I can even laugh (perhaps) at the memories, but then it was horrendous. How could a curate's wife, someone who gave talks about what a special blessing Lizzie had been to us, be capable of such awful anger and outbursts of frustration and rage? I was having to come to terms with the dark side of myself and I was finding it difficult.

It was harder to cope because I was constantly tired. Lizzie would always wake up by 6.30 a.m. and be in our bed, not still for a moment. On lighter mornings it would be earlier, 5.30 or 6 a.m. We could not snooze away while she occupied herself with toys, as she would probably be making a dough with cotton wool and cream that she had obtained from my dressing-table. Or she would play with my lipstick, or the loo roll from the bathroom, or a book which she would write all over and tear.

I so wanted to have a time to pray and read the Bible when I woke up but it was hard to concentrate. Unfortunately I needed a lot of sleep.

Having to be constantly on the alert became wearing when I took the children round to play with friends. Unless the door of the downstairs room was shut, Lizzie would be upstairs shredding loo paper, eating haemorrhoid cream or washing the bathroom floor with a flannel. Despite my friends always saying 'Oh she'll be all right', I could never relax and would weakly repeat, 'I'll just go and see what Lizzie is doing.'

Sometimes I was too late. If Lizzie drew with wax crayons, after two or three minutes she would start to eat them. Maybe it was just to get my attention, as the red or blue mouth naturally did. I would feel flattened, foolishly no doubt. For me, eating things was something toddlers did. Lizzie was still a toddler in many ways and I longed for her to grow out of that stage.

The best early morning escapade was one visit to Granny in Cornwall. Lizzie had clearly got up at about 5.30 a.m., before even Granny was up, and had opened the fridge, cracked an egg into a pot of cream and then drunk half the mixture.

The hour before tea-time every day continued to be difficult. I am always hungry and grumpy by 4.30 p.m. I was unable to watch the children while I cooked the supper because there was no room for them to play in the kitchen and the floor was cold and there was no hatch through to the living/dining-room. If I left any doors open, Lizzie would be upstairs wreaking havoc or hurting Nick, so Mark had to look after them. If he couldn't be there I found it difficult. There were many burnt saucepans, as I left the cooker to sort out the children.

I often felt angry with Mark because I envied him the freedom to go out and do his job on his own. I couldn't leave the mess and the fighting. I often felt angry with myself and my inability to cope, then I got angry with him—even though Mark did what he could to help me.

Part of the difficulty of Mark working from home was that he was present but not available. Sometimes in desperation I would shout into the study for Mark to help me. By then I was cross because I hadn't managed to cope on my own. I felt guilty at interrupting Mark, yet angry. I was a failure on every count. I projected my anger onto Mark and there was conflict between us.

All in all, much combined to make me feel sad and depressed. At the end of January I decided to try planning activities to do each day on a weekly cycle, so that I had an aim while playing with Lizzie. I would do cutting out, jigsaws, colour-matching one day, and other activities on other days. It helped me feel I was covering other things than the speech-oriented Portage activities.

By the middle of February I was so desperate about Lizzie continually scratching Nick on his face when my back was turned that I decided to talk to my neighbour. She and her whole family were very involved in our church, and I decided to ask her to pray with me about the scratching. I should have gone before, but I wasn't too ready to admit to outsiders that anything was difficult in those days.

I walked out of our front door, down the path, and rang the bell on the familiar light-oak door. 'Please be in,' I breathed. The door opened. 'Jean, can I talk to you for a bit? Could we pray about Lizzie?' Jean was always happy to pray with me. I was glad she was there. Two days later I took Lizzie to nursery school as usual. Nick was most reluctant to come

47

out, as usual wanting to play too, and I struggled to remove him from the Wendy house. As I did so, Lizzie's educational psychologist walked in. I had never seen her at the nursery before.

She saw Nick's face, covered with scratches, and asked how it happened. When I explained, she made an appointment to come round and plan a strategy to deal with the problem. I felt our prayers were already being answered.

When Lynn came, she suggested that I left Lizzie and Nick alone for one minute, three times a day, to start with—stressing how nice it was for brothers and sisters to be kind to each other. If no scratching occurred, I should praise them when I returned.

I found that, gradually, I could increase the time I left them and the scratching became less of a problem over the next few months.

I could have phoned for help but sometimes things don't seem bad enough to bother someone else with, or perhaps I didn't like to admit I had a problem. Sometimes behaviour seems inevitable and we don't realize it can be changed.

In January, the 'Educational Visitor', a liaison person in our area between school and home for under-fives, told us that we needed to have Lizzie 'statemented'.

The 1981 Education Act recognized that children with special needs should be integrated into mainstream education, as far as local authorities' economic policy would allow. In practice this could mean that where a large amount of money was already invested in special schools, support for children in mainstream education would be low in priority. Each child was supposed to be 'statemented'. A document or statement was produced to set out the special needs of the child and indicate how those needs were to be met in the school—for example, how many extra hours of nursery-nurse support or support-teacher help was needed. The idea was to safeguard the child and ensure that their needs would be adequately met.

The fear in our minds was that if Lizzie was statemented

now, when she had only just started at the school, a long list of problems might be produced in order to get more staffing. The education department might be unwilling to finance the extra help and the head could then say the school was unable to teach Lizzie. She would then be forced into special education without ever having a chance to prove she could cope in mainstream.

Whether to send a child to mainstream or to special school is a big issue for parents of handicapped children. Some parents feel that their children need the more protected environment of a special school, with its higher staff/pupil ratio, in order to grow and develop. For others, the environment of the ordinary school with the provision of extra input in some form, provides the challenge they feel will stimulate their child into fulfilling their potential. Each child is different. Each family is different. But every parent wants the best for their child.

Problems arise when parents feel forced by Local Education Authorities to accept an arrangement that they are not happy with. It seems often to be the case that parents wanting their children to have a chance in mainstream are persuaded to accept something else. Parents do not always feel valued or listened to by the relevant authorities.

At this time there were often articles and letters from parents in the Down's Syndrome Association Newsletter, indicating the feeling that education authorities might say one thing but, because of economics, revert to the policy of sending all Down's children to special school, regardless of their ability or needs. The parents might sometimes sound a bit paranoid, but their feelings were often based on insensitive handling by education authorities.

I was frightened of being pushed into a process I had no control over. I realized that I found it hard to trust God about Lizzie's schooling because I subconsciously felt that the educational machinery was somehow out of his control too.

Lizzie's statement became a priority in my praying. If it was needed, I prayed that extra speech therapy or nursery

49

help would be available at her nursery school and that the head of special needs would be happy to supply it.

At this time Lizzie was on a temporary placement at her nursery school. In March I had a discussion with the headmaster and asked for her not to be statemented yet but to stay on a temporary placement at the nursery. I felt it would give Lizzie time to show she could cope and then perhaps we could proceed later. He agreed.

I was anxious about the situation because nothing was permanent and I found the insecurity difficult. I felt as if we were always on probation, seeking approval. Perhaps this hooked up memories from the past for me: moving lots of times, as a child; always being new, different; trying to belong and be accepted. Unaware of the roots of these feelings at the time, I found it a cause of anxiety.

It was a real struggle. I wrote in my diary, 'We don't need to fight for things for Lizzie.' We didn't want to be aggressive but we were persistent in our desire for the best for her.

By May, speech therapy had been arranged for Lizzie for one afternoon a week and in June we were allocated a Portage teacher with skills in speech development who was superb. By the July in which Lizzie was four-and-a-half, a decision was made to put off producing a statement until September. The process of statementing took several months and we wanted it to be done in time to have a place agreed at a local primary school for when Lizzie was five. So we felt caught between it being done too early and not giving her a chance to develop and it being done too late, so complicating or holding up her entry to primary school. But we seemed to be moving in the right direction.

We had to face the issue squarely. Lizzie might not be able to cope with mainstream school and need to go to special school. Despite our strong feelings that segregation on the basis of being labelled handicapped was unjust, we had to agree that segregation on the basis of need was sensible.

Perhaps Lizzie needed the extra input, the individualized programme of work, available in a special school. I vacillated

50

when she behaved badly. But Mark felt as I did: if Lizzie could cope with mainstream she should have a chance to go there. We would never know unless she tried.

I wrote in June, 'I still feel the need to teach Lizzie to read before she is really ready. Does this show that I have still not accepted her problems? I feel Portage puts too much pressure on me. Lizzie is OK if she likes doing things, but if she doesn't, nothing will get her to co-operate. It is so frustrating. One day she will be brilliant and co-operative and then for several days she will not want to co-operate over anything. I then begin to wonder if the good day was a mirage, a figment of my imagination.' It was then that I wondered if I was being unrealistic about mainstream and her ability to cope there.

'We have started to give her vitamin B6 (with our doctor's agreement) which seems to help her become more relaxed and happy, and she now sleeps until 7 a.m. each morning.'[1]

In July, when Lizzie was four I wrote, 'Lizzie has begun to say two and even three words together occasionally. She cuts with scissors and can write her name (except the 'e'). She seems to be making a lot of progress. I feel I need to let go and let her do what she can, without all the pressure. It is so hard to keep going through all the fits and starts and temperamental behaviour.'

I wrote later: 'I feel more open to the idea of her going to a special school if need be.' We felt perhaps the local special school might be best and we decided to book an appointment to visit. I told her nursery teacher what I had done and she said that, given six months, Lizzie might be all right in mainstream. She had made good progress and her language was growing. From September she was to have speech therapy twice a week.

Mark and I went to see the special school. We went, willing for Lizzie to go there in September if necessary. It was a large school, with an excellent reputation. It was fully equipped

1. There is a lot of debate about the effectiveness of vitamin therapy, and your doctor should always be consulted.

with speech therapy rooms, hydrotherapy pool, music areas. We were shown round all the classes and were then taken to the class Lizzie would be in. I felt they were very keen for her to start.

She would be in the class for four years. The children were a mixed age-group. They appeared to be playing the same games I was playing with Lizzie now. I couldn't help feeling that four years in the same environment would not be stimulating.

We talked as we drove away. We still wanted to pursue mainstream for Lizzie. Despite making this decision, I wrote in my diary: 'I felt it doesn't matter if Lizzie goes to special school now. Maybe I hadn't accepted her limitations enough and I do feel I've taken a step forward. Wishing very much for her to stay in mainstream may be a form of non-acceptance of her problems.'

Letting go seemed important. Letting go of Lizzie and of schools...

Learning to trust God is such a basic idea. We were being asked to do that in every new, unknown, situation. We were being asked to dare to say, 'Yes, you can handle it. You are in charge.' Growth is painful, sometimes it is a struggle in the dark.

Lizzie was changing me and she was making me face my own insecurities and my own frustrations.

I had struggled with potty training all that year. I often felt hopeless and depressed about it. Eventually we realized that her real problem was constipation. Her muscles were not strong enough to keep her regular unless she had a very high fibre diet. Later she was put on a daily dose of Lactulose which also acts as fibre, and this has helped her. But her constipation had caused cystitis through urine building up in her bladder. There was no room for it to leave and it then became infected. Her accidents were because everything built up, and then she had no control over things.

I had become depressed about the unpredictability of it all and the mess. Somehow I was never prepared fully when we were out. Or, if I was prepared, it would happen in the swimming-pool, when all our belongings were in the changing-room. There were numerous situations where I felt embarrassed by my own seeming incompetence. I looked a fool. I wasn't in control.

It began to feel essential to me that I made her sit on the loo, holding her very firmly, until she had performed. It was all right if I left her for one day but if she went for more than two days I knew that an unpredictable and horrid mess would occur when I was least prepared for it. I felt cruel holding her down, and yet I couldn't bear the thought of another accident. Often my efforts were successful, but I felt worried and upset by the force I had to use and the anger and rage I often expressed over the accidents that happened.

I knew it was irrational, but sometimes I felt she did it on purpose. I also felt angry with God. Perhaps it was the first anger I'd vocalized. I sometimes muttered to myself: Why did God let it happen? Why do I have to deal with this?

I didn't see at the time that I was creating a vicious circle. Lizzie must have seen and felt my anger; she was very sensitive to moods. She may have seen this as a way of getting my attention if she failed to receive the cuddles which I know I found harder to give. It was hard to cuddle someone I felt was making my life a misery, and yet she couldn't help it, and the conflict was impossible to sort out.

These feelings spilled over into other areas of my life. Since I had written *Elizabeth Joy* I had been asked to speak to various groups of people: midwives, mothers, church groups, school children, medical students. When I went to speak I wanted to say that I believed God had given us Lizzie, yet I felt such a hypocrite. I knew I shouted at her and wasn't always loving. I was standing up trying to be honest and yet also trying to be a 'success' as a parent of a handicapped child. What was the reality? How did I cope with the conflicts? How did I cope with the horrible person I found myself to be, underneath?

Coming to terms with difficulties and with our own limitations is always hard. I was often helped, or at least soothed, by putting on my boots and taking the children clomping down the footpath to the woods, five minutes from our door.

These woods and the lake had been a constant oasis of peace and quiet for us, with the rustle of the leaves and the crunch of the twigs. I knew every rut on the muddy path down to the lake and exactly where to avoid the boggy bits on the walk to the wooden bridge where we could play 'Pooh sticks'—dropping our twigs into the water on one side of the bridge, and seeing whose twig would come out first on the other. There were tree stumps that became space-ships as Nick grew older. There were ducks to feed and hiding-places to explore in the bushes.

There was ice on the lake in the winter and slippy, icy mud under foot. There were sections of grass to play ball on and mud to slip into. There was a stile to climb, and then the walk home across the park to the large fallen tree trunk, sawn in half lengthways, where the children always played buses.

Captured for ever in the photos of that year are the games we played in the woods, the jumping, the laughter, Nick the bus driver in his bright red anorak. Lizzie and Nick in their Postman Pat jumpers and wellies, feeding the ducks. The ever-changing colours, the buds growing and developing, the leaves falling, then sprouting. Ever-changing and yet an anchor. A peaceful place. Somewhere that didn't cost anything, that didn't involve a car journey. A place that created games for fertile imaginations and will always live, strong and firm like the trees, in my memory.

After a walk, when we came back tired but invigorated for tea, I always vowed that we'd go more often, that I'd encourage our children to appreciate natural things and try to turn away from instant entertainment and turning on the TV. Memory omits to record the fact that I had to carry Lizzie home from every walk and that sometimes she'd sit down and refuse to move when we'd just arrived at the lake.

And it omits the feeling of relief that I hated to acknowledge when the clock approached a children's TV slot and a diversion was provided from the activities I had encouraged them to do.

This summer of 'the terrible twos', when we had two children at the same stage, we did have a very happy camping holiday in Suffolk. It was a first for the children and they enjoyed the freedom of a good camp site with an adventure playground and plenty of grass to play on.

Despite the struggles of this year there were many good memories. Lizzie and Nick sitting by the fireplace at Granny and Grandpa's, sharing Smarties on Lizzie's fourth birthday—their love for each other glowing out of their faces. The party in our garden when Nick was two, everyone sitting on the grass round a large tablecloth spread with crisps, sandwiches, cakes... Mums and children, friends, puppet shows, Sooty in funny hats, swings, sleep. Lizzie and Nick, hand in hand, walking through the car park at Thorpeness, both with a shock of fair hair bleached by the sun, brown as berries and happy.

5
The Waiting Game

Refreshed and brown after our few days camping we spent a week in Sussex, returning for the same Christian holiday we'd been on the previous year. This year the highlight for us was meeting another family who also had a child with Down's Syndrome, about the same age as Lizzie. We found we had so many things in common.

Here Lizzie met 'The Clown Daddy', one of the children's helpers dressed up as a clown to welcome the children. As we drove into the school where the holiday was held, he gave them ice lollies. Lizzie immediately fell in love with him and followed him round throughout the holiday. When we got home he painted her a picture of a clown that still hangs on her bedroom wall.

It was a good week—a chance to see old friends and recharge batteries—and life began to improve. There were times when the children would play happily together. One day in the long holidays I felt strong enough to invite five extra children to play, mostly older than mine. I was even able to write a letter while they occupied themselves sorting out the dolls house and the books, and helping our two to join in.

I wrote in my diary, 'I am beginning to feel a new freedom. Nick and Lizzie organize games a bit now. If they are dressing up, Nick says, "You put this on, Lizzie." He's two. It is a beautiful sunny day today and the children didn't wake up until 8 a.m. It was bliss. I feel full of life and want to attack the garden, a rare feeling!'

I was still struggling with my feelings of resentment when

Lizzie asked for cuddles and wanted to be picked up all the time. By contrast, I found it so easy to love and cuddle Nick. I suppose Lizzie asked so much because she sensed my reluctance, and somehow knew I didn't cuddle her as much as Nick. I decided to cuddle and hold Lizzie much more, despite my contradictory feelings, and I found that she became more amenable.

I wrote in my diary, 'I know deep down that she feels rejected and jealous of Nick and needs reassurance, not high expectations of her performance! When will I learn!'

In fact, she was beginning to read short sentences at this time, out of a book of photographs of her friend Ann, which I had made for her. I looked after Ann for a couple of days every week after playgroup. Each picture had easy sentences I had written underneath. 'Ann likes milk.' 'Ann likes Mummy and Daddy.' I began to find that Lizzie would very happily read or practise other skills after Nick had gone to bed. To begin with her reading was rewarded by chocolate buttons, but she became so pleased about it herself that she didn't need them any more.

Lizzie was becoming less frustrated and bolshy: her speech was improving; she was successful at reading and was able to be more grown-up. The cuddles became spontaneous again, and in September I wrote: 'I find I give her more cuddles now, and not just because I think she needs it. I am less cross with her and she loves giving me a big hug and a kiss. She also asks not to wear a nappy when she goes to bed, so I put one on her later!'

I felt we had crossed some bridges.

I needed some medical checks in September: I wanted to have a third child. The traumatic time in hospital after I'd had peritonitis, when Nick was one, had made me afraid of becoming pregnant, of not being able to cope with a third child—even of dying in the process. Mark prayed with me about it, and that helped me to feel more peaceful.

The night before I went to the doctor I read this verse in my Bible: 'To him who by means of his power working in us is able to do so much more than we can ever ask for, or even think of: to God be the glory' (Ephesians 3:20). I had a gut feeling everything would somehow be all right—and maybe not just 'all right' but better than we could imagine. By the end of September, I thought I might be pregnant.

At the beginning of October Lizzie had an assessment with the educational psychologist. I always felt rather keyed up about these occasions, but it went well. The reports from her nursery teachers were very encouraging, her Portage record showed her development to be age four to five (her actual age), except for language which, as always, lagged behind in the three to four age-group. The speech therapy assessment suggested speech levels of between three-and-a-quarter and three-and-a-half years.

I had felt that the Portage checklist was rather a crude measure of mental age. I wondered, when I listened to Nick, if we were over-estimating Lizzie. His thinking and understanding seemed to be on a deeper and more complex level. If on paper the gap between her chronological age and developmental age seemed small, I had to admit that the gap must appear to widen as she got older.

Despite my reservations about checklists, everyone felt the best placement for Lizzie was for her to remain at nursery school until the following summer, when she would be five.

I had asked about the possibility of Lizzie attending the local primary school from Christmas onwards, entering in the term she was five, but I had been told that, although the headmaster would have been happy with her presence, the teacher currently in charge of the reception class would not. In fact she refused to teach her. I found it hurtful to feel someone could reject a person they had never met, for no apparent reason. It seemed very unjust, yet it also seemed sensible for Lizzie to stay on longer at nursery school and build upon the skills she was already developing there.

Later on in the Autumn the headmaster of her nursery school asked me to see him, to read a report he had compiled about Lizzie so that a statement could be started on her. He read out something which, I realized later, must have been based on reports dating back to June or July, about her poor language development and immature behaviour. I found it very discouraging. I sat on the edge of the chair in his office and he calmly read the report aloud. I didn't take in anything very positive, and I felt demolished. It seemed so easy to dismiss a small child's efforts with calm detachment.

I left the office near to tears, and looked hard at the pavement as I walked home. Somehow I was sharing in the rejection and suffering that was part of what has gone wrong in the world. Lizzie was innocent, yet was rejected. Christ too, was innocent and yet was rejected. Perhaps all suffering was partly caused by rejection. I felt I shared in that suffering that day. Yet I knew that suffering could make us more as God wanted us to be—could change us from within—and I needed to accept it in that way.

By the beginning of January Mark felt he had to do something about looking for a new job. His current job had been meant to last for three to four years and we were approaching the end of the three years.

I wrote in my diary: 'There seem so many uncertainties. I am pregnant; the baby is due in June. There is no job yet for Mark and no school for Lizzie. It is so hard to keep waiting. Yet tonight I had a rare treat. Our midwife friend has started babysitting for us once a month, so that I can go up to the parish church to the evening service. I find so often God speaks to me very clearly in a place where I go as a visitor rather than a clergy wife. I felt encouraged. Despite appearances to the contrary, I have begun to believe that God has got everything in hand. He really will do so much more than we can imagine.

'I feel happier about the children. At Christmas Granny made a nurse's outfit for Lizzie, with a real blue and red cape and a fob watch on the apron. Nick had a doctor's coat, with a set of real bandages and plasters in a red case. They have played for hours, listening to each other's hearts with the stethoscope carefully chosen by Grandpa. I even manage to have a few minutes in the mornings now, when I wake up, to read my Bible and pray while the children play. Life feels more civilized!

'Lizzie is talking more in little sentences of three to four words. She talks to her dolls as she plays with them, and to Nick. He is a perfect friend for her. He plays with her as no one else does and they obviously love each other a lot, despite the conflicts. They are becoming closer in "mental age" all the time, and as Nick grows older he finds he can stand up to Lizzie more. The "accidents" seem to happen less often, although Lizzie still wears a nappy at night.'

It was a cold and snowy winter and in the end the water froze solid on the lake. One Sunday afternoon Mark took the children for a walk right across the ice, with the ducks sliding on it too. The snow lay a long time.

At the end of January a friend of ours called in on her way to Wales. At lunch-time, after we'd said grace, Lizzie piped up, 'Pray, Yvonne, journey.' So we did. Lizzie had grasped already what prayers were for! If the car wouldn't start and I was fuming at the wheel, Lizzie would call out from the back seat, 'Pray Mummy.' It was salutary sometimes.

29th January
Lizzie had her assessment today. The important one for her statement. We waited in the play area at the Children's Centre until Lizzie was called in. This familiar room had just a few parents and children quietly playing, subdued compared with the play sessions when the slide would be out, and the igloo made of covered foam would be a favourite hiding- and jumping-place. I wondered if I'd be asked to accompany her or not. Sometimes she responds better if I'm not there. I didn't want to put her off. This time I was asked to join the educational psychologist in her office, I was relieved that they chose to use the McCarthy Developmental Test and not the Griffiths test. Lizzie has done the Griffiths test many times and I felt if she was bored with it she might not concentrate well.

Lynn was very kind and Lizzie responded. She drew a beautiful picture of Nick and was very co-operative. Her building skills and language responses were not very good, but her number answers were better than I'd expected. The results as I remember them were: *Number related questions*: age 4; *Drawing*: 4yrs 9mths (her chronological age); *Bricks*: 2yrs 6mths; *Language*: 3yrs 2mths; *Picture-Matching*: 2yrs 9mths.

We drove off in the car, relieved that the ordeal was over. I felt Lizzie had done herself justice.

Since the beginning of the year Lizzie had made progress regarding her bladder and bowel control. For some weeks now Lizzie had been taking 10ml Lactulose Syrup daily (which acts like fibre in the gut) and this had helped with the accidents and constipation. I felt relieved that the conflicts and upset caused might be mostly a thing of the past.

March was a bad time. I was six months pregnant by now, I had 'flu and a cough which kept everyone awake. Mark's Mum was very ill. A baby died in the parish. I felt that God hung on to us and stopped us going under. It was very difficult—and then it was April, and still the endless waiting and wondering what would happen for Lizzie with schools.

I phoned the Special Education Department and was told that there would be a committee meeting in June to review their policy for Down's children in mainstream schools, so they couldn't give me any information until July.

If we moved, we were told, a new Local Education Authority would not accept a statement from somewhere else. We would need photocopies of all the reports and would have to start the process again. I didn't feel we had got anywhere.

Life continued as usual for the children. Their new climbing-frame was much enjoyed. Lizzie swung along the catwalk with help and I hoped it would help her chest to expand and help with breathing. Nick had fun too. There were our regular walks to the woods as the weather improved.

The children began to be more interested in the insects and fishing with sticks became popular.

Lizzie's fifth birthday was a windswept day which we decided to spend at the Tower of London. It was a grey day, grey like the buildings overshadowing the grassy areas where Lizzie walked past the ravens. A Topsy and Tim book about the Tower of London, a great favourite with the children, had precipitated the outing.

The photo of Lizzie and Nick with the Beefeater and the soldiers and the ravens, captured the traditional trappings of the place. But Lizzie was entranced by the crown jewels, the gold and silver in their brightly-lit cases. She had to be carried most of the way—we always forgot her low capacity for walking unless she had a great incentive. I found the climb to the top of the White Tower rather hard work myself, with only two months to go until the baby was born.

Lizzie had just a few friends to her party. It was a happy time. I often realized too late that a small party that I could cope with was much happier than a huge, riotous affair.

On 1 May I wrote in my diary: 'Lizzie is being difficult again. I got very angry about it today. She won't stay in her car seat in the car. She undoes the straps. On long journeys it can be dangerous with her rolling about in the back and trying to get in the front. She is grumpy and angry and refuses her lunch and wants to be fed. Perhaps it's because we have a trainee nursery-nurse placed with us for one afternoon a week. She helps Lizzie with reading and writing while I take Nick to toddler club. Magda makes Lizzie work very hard, maybe it's tiring her out.'

Looking back I can see that Lizzie was unhappy, and maybe worried that I didn't take her to toddler club—a group I ran at our church. Perhaps the pressure put on her to work was too much. At the time, I don't think I saw the connection with her regression. It was easy to fail to treat Lizzie like any other sensitive child, because she couldn't express her feelings and perhaps was less aware herself of what made her upset. But perhaps, also, I was still too obsessed with her learning to read and write to allow her to let her true feelings surface. I was too quick to interpret her bolshiness as irrational naughtiness, rather than a natural response to her situation.

10 May
The health visitor made a surprise call the other day. She doesn't often come but this time persuasively suggested that I should approach another local primary school as a place for Lizzie. She was keen that I should visit the school. So I went. I was delighted by the warm and positive reception from the headmistress. She would be pleased to take Lizzie if the Local Education Authority agreed.'

I wrote requesting a place from the person in charge of mainstream education. I realized through this incident that it is better to approach the school first, rather than the Local Education Authority. We could have waited for months before hearing anything positive otherwise. It is up to the head whether or not they wish to have a statement for a child. If they are prepared to take a child without a statement they can.

On 25 May Nick had his third birthday. It was a warm, dry day and we had about twenty children in our long garden sitting on the grass round a tablecloth spread with food. My parents came to help, as it was only a week before the baby was due. I made a simple teddy bear cake. It was not very professionally iced, but Nick liked it. The following weekend my parents came back to help me prepare for the birth of our third child.

The baby was due on the 10 June. The birth had been imminent for three weeks and I was getting very frustrated.

On 10 June we saw the head of Special Education. We were early, and walked up and down the High Street looking in the slightly run-down shops before being ushered into the offices. His opening words were, 'We can't make a definite decision today, of course.' He went on to talk at length about things I thought could have been said in a few minutes.

It seemed as if he was stalling, hedging. He knew what we wanted. But he wouldn't be open about it. It was humiliating.

In fact we thought Elizabeth would go to the school we had approached most recently. She would go without a statement, but with support from the special school and some nursery help. So now we needed a letter of confirmation. Nine months seemed a long time to wait to get this far and not be quite sure, still, where Lizzie was going. And there were still no jobs for Mark...

That evening a small group met in our sitting room to pray. And suddenly I was set free from my feelings of anger and frustration. I was able to express my love to God. I knew that he was able to bring the baby in his time, and sort everything else out, when he wanted to. I could 'take my hands off'. I remembered the words, 'Be still and know that I am God.' I needed to let God be God. I'd not had this kind of struggle before when I was pregnant, but both the other children had come early.

I had very much wanted another girl, but I realized, as we prayed, that I didn't mind any more. We couldn't dictate to God. This baby was his gift to us, boy or girl, whole or handicapped. Peace enveloped me, a peace that would carry me through the next few days. God knew what I needed.

Four days later, Susannah Ruth was born, at four in the morning, weighing 8lbs 3oz. With her birth, I sensed that our family was complete in every way.

Inside her birth-card we wrote the verse that had meant so much to me: 'To him who is able to do so much more than we ask or think, to God be glory.' On the front, under a picture of a rainbow, were the words, 'What he promises, he performs.'

6
Susannah

Susannah's was the happiest and least stressful of all the births for me. The week at home resting afterwards with my Mum helping with the children leaves a rosy glow of memories... Gradually the soreness wore off, the muscles slowly returned to normal, and life began again. Feeding went well: she was a peaceful, happy baby.

I wrote after Susie was born: 'I cried a bit for Lizzie after Susannah arrived. Having Susannah made me realize I loved Lizzie in a special way. She has become more special since Susannah's arrival. She's been very helpful and grown-up about helping to look after her. Lizzie has had one completely dry night so far. It is fanciful, I know, to suppose she is showing me she is my "big" daughter.'

Susannah had a positive effect on Lizzie but Nick found it hard. He was really ill with tonsillitis for the two weeks after Susie's birth. Was it a subconscious protest? A fear of rejection? He had been replaced...

30 June
We received a letter from the Education Department today. Lizzie is able to go to our local primary school—the one where the teacher refused to have her in September, despite the head's encouragement.

Just after Susie was born I had gone to see this headmaster again—the school was much nearer than the one which had offered us a place. With Nick at a next-door playgroup it was much more sensible for Lizzie to go there. I wondered if the headmistress of the other school had prodded him into action. He said he'd reorganized the teachers. The reception class teacher would be willing to have Lizzie. There were vague offers of extra help from the Education Department. I was overjoyed.

Yet all through this year of trying to find a place for Lizzie, again and again I felt the unfairness of having to beg as a big favour for my child to go to our local school, when all other children—by virtue of being 'normal', regardless of whether they were co-operative or even very bright—automatically had a right to go.

I felt like an intruder.

At nursery school, especially to start with, there was always the threat: 'If she isn't good enough, she will have to leave.' It was only a 'temporary placement'. It wasn't said by anyone, but every assessment seemed not just an assessment of my child, but an assessment of me. Had I worked hard enough to make Lizzie 'acceptable'?

I knew other parents of handicapped children felt the same. It seemed ironic to me that at the same time as parents of 'normal' children were allowed to send their children to the school of their choice, provided there was a place, we had to beg on bended knee for our children to be given a chance to try. Many 'normal' children had behavioural problems or learning difficulties, but my impression was that they were allowed to start off in mainstream education. For handicapped children, various assumptions were made about their level of ability before they were given the opportunity to develop at all.

We felt as if we were taking on a system of bureaucracy and risking 'disapproval' and the label 'unrealistic' or 'demanding', or—worse—'difficult parents', for insisting on giving our children a chance.

As far as Lizzie's place was concerned we had not pushed, but we stuck to our guns and went through all the correct procedures. We had come, in the end, to the conclusion that it was better for Lizzie not to have a statement for the present. We had to trust the promise of extra help, even though it was only a promise. I was simply delighted Lizzie could start, and I looked forward to September and her first day at full-time school.[2]

11 July
Lizzie was sitting in a deckchair under a tree in the garden today, with the sun pouring through, making patterns on her. 'Me speckled,' she said. She told her doll to 'stop that annoying noise', and 'I'm joking' came out after something that she had said. I hadn't expected that someone who finds it hard to express herself in words, should have so many descriptive and funny things she wants to say.

At last I've found someone who can cut Lizzie's hair in a pretty, modern style, who didn't give up after the first three cuts. She just didn't accept Lizzie's reluctance to sit still and co-operate. In the past I've had to cut her hair myself, and it's not looked very professional. I'm relieved. It's seemed hard to get Lizzie to look really nice. I have even felt guilty that perhaps she didn't look as nice as she might and people would feel I hadn't tried. There I go again! I still seem to find things to feel guilty about.

Lizzie left nursery school today. I'll miss the other mothers I've got to know. Lizzie will certainly miss 'Hartley' and 'Fewell', as she calls her teachers, and 'my children'. I think of her there with her special day badge on (a plum), going to the TV room to watch 'You and Me', and writing in her special book. She has spent two years at the nursery.

It has been a time of successful integration, she speaks to all the teachers now—she didn't when she started. She tries quite long conversations and I'm sure her progress is partly due to hearing other children talk all day, and being in the encouraging, warm environment of that particular school.

2. *The policy of statementing children who are in mainstream schools varies from Education Authority to Education Authority. Local Management of Schools may affect statementing policy in the future.*

A letter came to tell us that an extra welfare assistant had been appointed for Lizzie, for the new school. Everything has worked out for the best. I've been reading a book about another mother's experience of teaching her Down's child to speak. It's brought back my old fears of not working hard enough with Lizzie, the anxiety that if I had done more, perhaps she'd be better at speaking. But this time I've realized what is going on.

Lizzie is not the same as another child. She doesn't have to be. It is not a competition, or a race to get anywhere first. Our whole family matter, not just Lizzie's progress in speaking. I'm sure I do not need to be threatened so much by other people's achievements, to feel they automatically make me a failure. I know this in my head. I still have to work hard at making my feelings fit in with what I believe.

Yet I really do feel it doesn't matter any more. She is happy. She can speak, even if it is only in short sentences. She says what she wants to: 'Baby crying', 'Don't want to', 'I'm are' (for 'I am'), 'Me do it.' If she thinks Daddy is laughing at her she says 'Don't mock.' Lizzie is very keen to be understood and appreciated and is very upset if she isn't. She is very possessive of Susannah in church and fends off other children from the carrycot perched on the pew.

She is on and off about her reading. It's holiday time and the children often ask to play 'playgroups', so we do some writing and reading. I'm hoping Lizzie has got enough grounding to keep up at school to start with, and to be encouraged to keep working. I don't know how the breaks and lunch-time will work out yet, though. Will Lizzie behave or try to run away?

On holiday I had cause to ponder on the benefits of having three children when one is handicapped. For me, Susannah has put Lizzie and Nick in perspective. No longer is Nick 'the normal child', of whom so much is expected, and Lizzie the handicapped one. They are all just brother and sisters.

By this time I felt I was able more and more to let go of Lizzie and not force her to work, nor worry so much if she didn't. I was learning not to try to make her 'normal' any more. She was thriving on being free to play imaginary games with Nick in the garden, going to bed, getting up, being in a space-ship... and watering the plants. I was only doing reading when she asked and I tried to play some games from 'Reading through play'—games that involve reading in order to play the games. That worked quite well.

I love reading to the children and I wanted to make plenty of alternatives for them instead of just turning on the television for instant entertainment. We read modern versions of Bible stories, which the children loved, as well as a wealth of beautiful children's books, supplied by raiding the library. It sometimes took an effort to get out the paints and Play-Doh and not turn on the telly...but it was worth it.

Susannah was a happy little girl, and I took positive pleasure in the pretty clothes she'd been given. I felt sad when I decided to sell the pram which I didn't really use. Then I took her first baby clothes, the cradle and bath to a friend who needed them for her baby. I had to nerve myself to get rid of these things, yet it was right to move forward into a new phase. Our family was now complete.

21 August
Lizzie wrote her name on her own for the first time today. She has traced it over dots for more than a year, which shows she has to be very confident before she will do something new. She also cut out shapes and stuck them on some paper. We made sock puppets, and Lizzie and Nick went on a long 'pretend' visit to the seaside inspired by 'Playschool'.

I finished *Jacob's Ladder* by Jan Lloyd today. It's the story of a Down's child learning to talk. But every situation is different. It is no good simply trusting to systems or methods or people. It is not a competition to see how bright we can make our Down's child. It is easy to slip back into feeling that it is. But the book has encouraged me to make sure Lizzie's learning is generalized into other areas. In the past I've often been so keen to prove she could do something that I thought one attempt at it was enough... We practised some sorting and classification games yesterday—size, shape and colour. The book has also made me aware that we may be entitled to more than five hours' extra welfare help a week in school. Jacob had twenty hours', and five hours' extra teaching time, but everywhere is different.

In the past I've often felt threatened or condemned by other people's stories. But now I don't. Perhaps I'm really accepting the differences—and accepting myself at last.

Yesterday Lizzie changed Susannah's nappy all on her own. I had taken Susie upstairs and laid her on our bed, when the phone rang. I left her upstairs with Lizzie, hoping she would come to no harm. When I got back, I found the wet nappy taken off and on the floor. Lizzie was carefully spreading cream on Susie's bottom from my perfume creme pot! She had chosen a set of clean clothes for her, all lined up ready. I had to laugh. Apart from the rash that appeared the next day, no harm seems to have been done. How much Lizzie absorbs by watching people!

4 September
I had a great sense of pride and joy as Lizzie walked confidently into school in her uniform today. She had a three-inch hem on her dress, as she was the smallest in the class. But she looked very smart in her blue-checked dress and her blazer.

My delight was tempered, however, as the days passed and Lizzie was unco-operative, refusing to do things for the teacher or the extra welfare assistant. The lunch-breaks were a long period of unstructured time for Lizzie. She kept running into school to get pens and pencils to do something. Could she take things to do? Should she come home to lunch? The educational welfare assistant, because of limited transport, could come to school on only two weekday mornings, rather than for one hour a day, so it was not an ideal arrangement. But I liked her teacher.

By 1 October I could write: 'Lizzie seems to be slowly learning. I feel happy seeing her run out more confidently from school at the end of the day. I have to admit that the day is peaceful at home! There is less fighting, but I miss Lizzie too. To start with, I felt a bit insecure—I was no longer in charge of helping Lizzie to learn. I tried to play some games when she got home, to make up for it, but I soon realized she would be exhausted. So we stopped, and she now comes home to watch television or listen to stories. It's hard not being able to monitor her progress myself—to let go.'

At the end of October I saw the headmaster, to review how Lizzie had got on at school in the first half-term. She had wet and dirtied her pants a lot. The welfare assistant wanted to leave at Christmas. It seemed hard because, for a Down's child, Lizzie had done so well. Yet in a normal school it didn't appear like that.

At half-term we decided to take advantage of the fact that Mark's brother was working in Paris. We found a very cheap ferry deal and drove over to visit.

We had an exciting five days, visiting all the famous places, reminding ourselves of the hugeness of the galleries and staircases at the Louvre. We also saw something of Parisian suburban life, as my sister-in-law introduced us to puppet shows and donkey rides in the local park, and the delights of the local patisserie.

Poor Lizzie found it all too much. The disturbance to her routines, the strange language, and late nights travelling led us sadly to feel, as we returned home, that perhaps it would have been better for Lizzie to have stayed with my parents.

Nick had delighted in the novelty of a different culture and longed to return. For Lizzie, it was too confusing and alien. Her way of protest was to ask to be carried all the time, and to sit down and wait—and scream—in the middle of the Louvre or a strange route to the metro. These were not the happiest moments in an otherwise special week.

It was sad to feel she'd have been happier at home—yet we were being realistic and admitting her limitations. Perhaps that was a good thing. We want to treat Lizzie as normal in every way, yet she does have special problems. It isn't wrong to acknowledge those. In the past I would probably have seen this admission as failure on our part—now it just seems sensible.

Lizzie is always happiest with a gentle relaxed routine, in a place that she knows. However, when she does have a break from normal everyday life, she returns to it stimulated and ready to make progress.

18th November
The Bishop of Lichfield has asked Mark to be vicar of a parish in the Black Country. We went to see the place last Friday. We stopped looking in *The Church Times* for jobs every week sometime back. We decided to wait until someone phoned us, or asked us to go and look at a job. When the phone call came, it was from an area we'd never thought of going to. But we'd put it in God's hands, so we had to follow it up.

Mark visited the parish after a clergy conference—it was conveniently placed on the route home. He felt excited by this job. We went there together on a cold, murky, November day. We saw Victorian houses lining the streets and industrial buildings scattered across derelict land—an unfamiliar landscape of flats and houses, canals and pubs.

The enormous old vicarage was scheduled to be replaced by a modern one, to be built in the garden. I baulked at the high ceilings and the huge bedrooms—how could we heat it, let alone furnish it? We stepped out into the garden—and then I relaxed. It was a wonderful garden, full of trees, and surrounded by an old Victorian wall—an oasis in an urban environment. We were being given special help to make this move.

Easter seemed the right time for the move. We were sad to leave our friends, but it was right for us to move on.

The matter of schools was a great concern to us—and I telephoned the local school in our new parish.

Heart beating fast, I asked the $64,000 question. 'I am enquiring whether you would be prepared to take my daughter Elizabeth: she has Down's Syndrome.' There was no pause or hesitation. The headmistress simply said 'You've made my day.' She would be pleased to have Elizabeth. She had worked with Down's children before, and did some of the remedial work herself. Nick could start at nursery school at Easter and would be full-time in September. I knew he was ready for school, although he'd be only four.

I replaced the phone and jumped up and down with delight. I couldn't quite believe it. The very problem we had struggled so hard with was solved in a few minutes' telephone conversation. No doubt because Lizzie was already in mainstream education it was easier to transfer her without red tape, and she had no statement. But it was more than that. For someone to be so positive about having her at school was a tonic to me, and a very clear confirmation of our decision to accept this job.

It is so like God to use the things that we struggle with to bless and encourage us. Again Lizzie had proved to be God's signpost for us. And his timing is perfect. When we told the headmaster about the move he was pleased because he admitted he had been concerned about Lizzie moving into a bigger class...which would have happened at Easter.

That same day Nick was offered a nursery place for January, but I decided he should stay on at his playgroup until we moved. Yet I felt a little sad that Nick wouldn't go to the lovely nursery school Lizzie had been to, and that he'd reluctantly left each day for the past two years—longing to stay himself.

We went to visit our new home once more before we

moved—to measure up for curtains and also to be shown the plans of the new vicarage by the architects.

On this visit Susannah seemed ill. It wasn't a usual kind of illness. She cried at the bright lights on the motorway; she had a temperature and slept a lot, and she began to make peculiar jerking movements. I began to get worried.

Three weeks later I was desperate to get a proper medical opinion. The jerks were worse, but no one took it seriously. Fortunately—providentially—Lizzie had to visit the pediatrician at the Children's Centre for a check-up. When the doctor saw Susie she rushed her in for an emergency admission. Susie was having what were called 'Salam attacks'. If they continued there was an 80 per cent chance of brain damage. I felt shattered. She could develop epilepsy...she could be brain damaged...

I drove her to the hospital and we were admitted to the children's ward. They had to observe the fits to start with, then arrange a brain scan and an electro-encephalogram to measure the pattern of Susannah's brain waves. Electrodes were stuck onto her head and I held her tight as a print-out recorded a mass of waves—even I could see that the pattern looked uneven and disjointed. The following day she was put on daily injections of a synthetic hormone that acted like steroids.

After about twenty-four hours the fits slowed down and then stopped altogether. After five days in hospital we were allowed home. Arrangements were made for a nurse to do the injections and we tried to get back to normal. Nick developed tonsillitis again on our return.

The drugs increased Susannah's appetite and reduced her sleeping times, so I was feeding her cereal in the middle of the night. She was seven months by now. It was a nightmare. Gradually the dosage was reduced and after six weeks she came off the drugs altogether. Then the waiting game began...the waiting to see if she had been damaged by this experience.

Everyone was praying for her. But I felt empty and

74

depressed. Had God brought us to this point only to let us down?

It seemed too much to bear. Once again, as when Nick was nine weeks old and had been hospitalized, our youngest child's life was threatened. And even when the fear of her death had gone, there was the possibility of brain damage. It seemed so hard. Lizzie was born as she was... But to have a perfectly normal child suddenly handicapped—damaged by a mysterious illness—was too hard to bear.

I found myself watching for problems with Susie's speech or walking...but she continued to develop. Just before we were due to move she had an assessment, as Lizzie had done. The pediatrician who had asked for her admission originally, tested her and was tearful with relief as she said there was no known damage. God had answered our prayers. Susannah was all right.

During Susannah's illness many friends had supported us—underlining our sense of belonging to the community we had to leave. I dreaded the separation—the kind of dying there is in moving...starting everything from new...but we had to go through with it.

In the last months before we moved I would take Lizzie to school each morning to this beautiful spot, often shrouded in mist as the winter days slowly moved towards spring. We'd crunch over the frozen ground and look at the golden ball of sun slowly edging its way up into the sky over the flats and buildings that mark the edge of London. Before us was the golf course where the children played in the summer, with the scarred burnt tree trunk pointing up to the sky.

I was sad that Lizzie would not always be coming here. Once again I couldn't belong to a community I would have loved to have been permanently part of. The school was a happy, lively place, full of good education, yet neither Lizzie nor Nick could be part of it. I would miss the friends we were making. The walks back home across the golf course, school bags trailing, happy voices; the cups of tea and the games at our friends on the corner, with their twin boys Nick's age and their daughter in Lizzie's class. We'd had fun together, tossing ideas around about children and life, moaning and rejoicing together—I would miss it all, despite the times when Lizzie had been grumpy because she'd been tired, or was aggressive, snatching toys, pulling hair and shoving people. But life is a mixture of joy and tears, laughter and sadness. I knew we could not hold on just to the good times but sometimes I wanted to, very much.

Lizzie's sixth birthday also happened to be her last day at the primary school, where she had begun her 'mainstream' career. The headmaster told us how remarkably well Lizzie had become part of the class, indistinguishable from the other children. Her class teacher had surprised me at a parents' evening by saying that she felt Lizzie was within the range of the class. After Christmas she had had a new teacher and a nursery-nurse who had come for five mornings a week and it had worked much better.

The head felt Lizzie could cope with mainstream school up to the end of juniors. He was very pleased with how it had turned out and felt it had been very successful.

The problems of the first few months had been gradually resolved; the toilet accidents were fewer. Lizzie had accepted the idea of school. So we hoped she could carry on in the same way in the new school.

The next two weeks were consumed by packing and on 21 April, in time for the new term, we moved to the Midlands. Following the removal van up the motorway, I cried for all we'd left behind, and for the unknown ahead. The children sat in the back, excited about the big new house...

7
A New Life Begins

The boxes were stacked up in the large red-curtained sitting-room, some half-unpacked. There seemed to be miles of corridors and landings, uncarpeted, along which we clattered as we tried to settle in. It felt strange to us to live in such a big house, without neighbours adjoining us.

We walked on the narrow, uneven pavements along the little streets to school on the first day of term, over the hump-backed bridge that crossed the canal, and past the tobacconist's into whose depths Lizzie would often disappear unannounced when she thought I should buy her some sweets.

I saw other parents taking their children to school. Inside the green railings we joined the throng of parents in the small playground. It was all so different here. Would I get used to it all? Yet I was attracted by the friendly smiles and chatter. It was hard for us to understand the local accent at first, but we felt welcomed.

Nick didn't want to stay, and for the first few weeks felt miserable and depressed. He missed his friend so much and his new classmates laughed at his southern accent. It was a month before he said, 'Oh good', when I said it was time to go to school.

Lizzie was welcomed immediately by mothering girls who took her under their wing. I felt we belonged, and no one made us feel we shouldn't be there. I didn't worry about how Lizzie would get on, although I felt sympathy for her new teacher with a large class to teach in the hall while they waited for new classrooms to be converted in another building.

Perhaps it was the enthusiasm and confidence of the headmistress that made my sense of inadequacy about Lizzie disappear almost overnight.

I was never made to feel that anyone was doing us a favour. Lizzie belonged here. She was welcomed and accepted. No one asked me about her as if she was a special case, and people were sympathetic but matter-of-fact in their approach.

Something underlay the atmosphere of this school that I had never found before. I began to realize that the headmistress and the staff had a commitment to the children that seemed rare. The headmistress also had a commitment to God that spilled out naturally in assemblies and in her dealings with people.

Before we had arrived, she had told the school about Lizzie and prepared them for her. She had stressed their need to treat her like everyone else and not to mother her. The book I had written had been bought and extracts read in assembly. I felt touched that such a special welcome had been given us. There seemed a kind of excited interest in getting to know Lizzie—and the mothering ceased pretty sharply when the 'mothers' realized Lizzie could stand up for herself. The odd kick on the shins went a long way in making her point.

There were others in the class who needed extra help, and at the beginning of the new school year a nursery-nurse was appointed half-time, to help Lizzie and a few others. Lizzie still had no statement but she had been provided with the help she needed.

The nursery-nurse had herself had a Down's child who had died at the age of two. A special bond developed between her and Lizzie during the two years that followed.

Life here was very different, there was no doubt. Occasionally I would panic and wonder whether we would settle in and adjust. We had left the safe shelter of the culture we had grown up in. But even in the panic there was a certainty that we were meant to be here. Not least in the way Lizzie settled at school and made such excellent progress.

As the first term purred to a sunny end, and the holidays approached, the children played in the garden with its bushes and hideouts. We lazed on the grass, delighted at discovering old friends who lived near enough to visit. They sustained us in the initial isolation and strangeness, and surrounded us with familiarity.

We discovered the delights of the local life museum, a walk away. We took our friends to see it. We explored the beautiful countryside and historic towns and the animal park where we first saw real live badgers.

Our camping holiday was spent in nearby Wales, after an idyllic journey through mountain passes, stunning in their unfamiliarity. Apart from punctures, and stalling on steep hills, we loved our exploration of that wet and misty land. The beaches backed by mountains, the castles and the water combined to bewitch us and draw us back again.

In those months of early vulnerability, on holiday we found more old friends in unfamiliar territory and knew we might never have come there unless we'd moved to the Midlands.

My sister, too, now lived near enough for us to visit, and her company helped us settle in.

The summer passed and excitement grew as the garden was fenced off and the new vicarage was begun. The foundations seemed to take months to grow. Then the structure of the house appeared. The roof was on by February and we began to feel we might really live there. Each weekend we would walk around the cement dusted boards, planning each room.

Lizzie was now in the top infant class, learning to copy words and progressing with her reading. Maths was always difficult but she made a number book and, during the year, her understanding of numbers up to ten slowly increased. Her new teacher helped to foster her love of Raymond Briggs' wonderful picture story, *The Snowman*. The class watched the video in the winter and Lizzie received a Snowman pillowcase for her birthday. The Snowman replaced Postman Pat as her passion.

There were no assessments. Once a year I was invited to see the educational psychologist to check there were no problems in her placement. It was very relaxed and informal.

The nursery-nurse came in the afternoons and helped Lizzie with creative work, painting and drawing, cutting and sticking. This arrangement changed in the following school year and she was able to help Lizzie with her maths and to use the sentence-maker to build her own sentences. Lizzie eventually progressed onto a word book.

First-year juniors, when Lizzie was eight, became a year of growth in many areas. C. S. Lewis's magical stories, *The Chronicles of Narnia* were first shown on television and Lizzie loved them. 'Edmund teases Lucy, Mummy. That's not fair!' Lizzie said indignantly. She understood that Aslan the lion represented Jesus and loved to watch our video recording of the series. We heard the tapes of the stories in the car and she drew pictures of Aslan on the stone table, about to die to save Edmund... It had touched her sensitive heart.

Christmas was a chance to buy Lizzie a small battery-powered organ. She loved it and improvised daily, always appearing like a concert pianist in her style although we wouldn't recognize the music. Lizzie would copy the outward form of a thing but did not grasp the heart. It began with her 'rubbish' writing that eventually grew into real words. It continued with her 'reading' of books. She could not read the actual words, but little phrases like 'the blue, blue sea...' would come from behind an open book.

Eventually, in the second year of juniors, when Lizzie was nine, she learnt to play Jingle Bells on her organ at an after-school club, the keys colour-coded with stickers. She was delighted. It was in that year too that she began to join in the singing lessons at school, and sang the words in time to the music.

Her best friend was keen to play the drums and they

enjoyed a special friendship. They played on equal terms. He wasn't hurt by Lizzie's rude and grumpy behaviour, when she was tired after school. He seemed unperturbed when she ignored him and decided to watch the television instead. He walked home with her, hand-in-hand, always on the same wave-length.

During the first two years I wasn't able to do very much work at home with Lizzie. She had separated school and home into neat compartments. Any workbooks I happened to have she refused to touch with a barge-pole, despite gentle encouragement from school to try anything I wanted. But the separation existed. It was as if she said, 'This is home, Mummy—I don't do that kind of thing here.' So I gave up. For the first time I wasn't closely involved in her learning, and I felt totally happy about it. We did very little except hear her read her school reading-book each night. She was reluctant to do that—until this last year (three years after our move).

PART TWO

LIZZIE AND HER LIFE TODAY

'My times are in your hands.'

Psalm 31, verse 15

*The road stretches out,
and as I take
one step,
and two, the road moves on*

*No end in sight.
Just new
horizons.
But you are there,
taking the steps
as I take them.
Sharing
the adventure.*

*Lord, it's risky.
There's so much space.
But the
real shelter is not in the walls I build.
It's in you.*

Eddie Askew, from *Alive to God*

8

Lizzie and School

Just a few months ago, I realized I hadn't checked Lizzie's progress against the Portage checklist, for about a year. I had assumed that since she was now eight, she would have passed the items for age five–six but when we looked I discovered some areas that still needed help.

Lizzie decided that she loved her special time with Mummy after Susie had gone to bed and while Nick did something else with Daddy. It was like old times. When she was younger, I'd found that Lizzie was bright and alert just before bedtime. We practised reading, learning the days of the week and tying shoelaces.

Perhaps it was the special attention that made her enjoy it so much, but she was also so much more confident about her reading that she would grasp the story as she read it, and she seemed to enjoy it.

Perhaps there is a watershed with learning to read, beyond which life becomes easier. I began to feel that maybe Lizzie was passing it now. It seemed to lie somewhere around level 4 of Ginn 360 in Lizzie's reading scheme!

This school year, the second in the juniors, began without Lizzie's special beloved nursery-nurse. I was apprehensive to start with, and I felt that Lizzie too was worried about who would help her.

The headmistress had felt it was time Lizzie was weaned from her special help, so that she could become more independent and take her place as an ordinary member of the class. The transition occurred. The head's confidence was rewarded. Lizzie coped. One day we had to go for a hearing test. I went to the classroom to collect Lizzie and found her seated at her table ready for a spelling test. She had written the date at the top of the page.

Lizzie was there just like everyone else. I suddenly realized what a long way she had come. It reminded me of a visit made to the school by a new school nurse in the previous year. 'Is there something wrong with that child?' she had innocently asked at the end of her visit to the class. 'There was just something that made me wonder.' She hadn't noticed that Lizzie had Down's Syndrome. 'Just a bit,' said the head, and recounted the tale to me with glee, later in the day.

This term a new nursery-nurse has joined the staff in the afternoons to help with practical work. But she is shared with the other children and the advent of the National Curriculum means that extra help is invaluable.

Lizzie's independence seems firmly established. She goes back to the classroom to collect her reading book if she has forgotten it. She waits in the playground to go into school with Nick on the mornings I have to teach. She remained in a dance class on the first visit, with Nick and a friend, while I popped out to the shop. These are all things she would never have attempted a year ago.

Very occasionally she still has 'accidents', but the last one was due to the fact that the button on her trousers was very stiff, and she didn't ask for help. She is sometimes still not confident about asking for help from her teacher or others, but her confidence is growing and her self-respect with it.

In front of a crowd she becomes nervous. In a recent assembly she was word-perfect at the rehearsal, but sat down mute at the performance. At least she now joins in the songs.

There has been only one incident of bullying by others. Lizzie was pushed into the outside toilet, her glasses were pulled off, and the bully threatened to smash them. This happened about three times, much to Lizzie's distress, before complaints to the teachers and the parent concerned put a stop to it.

I was never sure that the bullying had anything to do with the fact that Lizzie has Down's Syndrome. She sticks up for herself very forcibly, is well able to kick and pull, and exerts great strength. I suspect it was much more likely she was bullied because she is a girl and wears glasses, and because she is rather short.

As Lizzie has grown older, her aggressive streak is less apparent and she seems to relate better to her friends. One girl came round after school and spent hours going through the dance routines Lizzie would need to know at her dance class, to help her settle in to her first lesson. (She then accompanied Lizzie to the class and danced next to her.)

Lizzie's art developed last year, under the able tutorship of the headmistress who looked after Lizzie's class for two terms. She painted a lovely picture of an owl on a branch above a nest of eggs. And she made a life-size model of the 'armour of God', originally for assembly. This now hangs on her bedroom door, frightening anyone who, unaware of the silver foil that gleams in the moonlight, takes a midnight trip to the loo.

The owls were the result of the special interest in wildlife fostered by the headmistress. One day in the summer term the whole class took overnight bags and set off by coach to a local nature reserve and camp site. Lizzie had packed her bag the night before, excited at her independence. In the past she'd often packed a bag to go and stay downstairs in the playroom, as part of an imaginary game. This time it was for real.

Lizzie had never been away on her own before. I waved a little anxiously from the roadway. Lizzie didn't notice me: she was engrossed in talking to her friends. We wondered how she would cope with the walking, but she managed it most of the time (although she often shows reluctance to walk far with us). I forgot to pack a nappy for her. She was still not dry at night. But I needn't have worried. They all returned safely the next day, Lizzie apparently so excited she hadn't gone to sleep until midnight. She was so tired when she came home that it took about three days for us to find out how she had got on.

The headmistress had taken her to the loo at 3 a. m. She had had her first dry night ever. We realized that with a bit of dedication on our part we might be able to climb this hurdle too—one that had stumped us for eight years.

Lizzie loves school. Dinner times are no longer the problem they were when she began her school career. She plays pop bands with her best friend and Nick in the playground.

She is almost always the last to come out of school, escorted by her teacher. One day she worried everyone by running out of the school gate on her own. She hasn't done it since. She used to rush up to the railings and swing on the gate. She does that less now. She always takes her coat off when she sees me and expects me to carry it home, even if it is freezing cold. Her classroom is hot and Lizzie doesn't sweat. It is the only way she has of cooling off after a hard day's work.

I understand now why she sometimes undressed in public places when she was little. It was embarrassing for us—but she must have been hot and felt like letting off steam, although she couldn't tell us at the time. So many of her actions which once seemed meaningless, now that we understand, take on a significance and show that there was a logical person behind the speechless toddler. If only we'd been able to believe it.

We meander slowly up the road, schoolbags trailing. If we can avoid the supermarket where Lizzie wants to rush in and swipe a bag of crisps, begging me to pay for them, we can walk home.

She is more willing about the half-mile walk now, negotiating the pavements with more care and awareness, waiting at the numerous kerbs ready to cross.

Soon she'll be learning how to go to the corner shop on an errand. She and Nick have tried it once or twice with me following some yards behind. Lizzie is growing up. School has played a tremendous role in developing her self-confidence and helping me to relax and believe she will do well. I feel sure too that it has helped her language to develop to a point at which she can say anything she wants to, although she finds some words difficult to articulate.

We are grateful for the headmistress's acceptance and belief in Lizzie, and for the staff who work hard to help her. We are grateful to God for bringing us to this place. It is here that we have become part of a normal community. Lizzie goes to school with the others. We are not separated by a bus that takes her miles away.

Integration really has worked for Lizzie so far. She has real friends, she is learning and progressing. She may not have had allowances made for her, she may not have had as much individual teacher time as in a special school, but I feel that Lizzie's place at our local school has enabled all of us to have confidence in her. And it's given Lizzie confidence in herself.

Each child is different. What works well for one may not work for another. But in our case Lizzie has been accepted and liked for herself. As a family we are no different from any other. Why should we be, just because one of our children has a problem? Families who are cut off from the community they live in, because their child is bussed elsewhere, must suffer a kind of isolation that underlines their difference. It must be particularly hard if they have no other children at the local school. It may be the only solution for the education of their child, but why should they be isolated in the process? There are no easy answers—unless more schools will accept children with special needs.

What of the future?

In the immediate future there is the school's performance of 'Joseph's Amazing Technicolour Dreamcoat'—a musical version of the Bible story of Joseph. Lizzie is in the dance group as one of Joseph's brothers. But what of the longer term?

When Lizzie started at primary school, the head told us he

thought she could cope until the end of Juniors. Now we want to pursue the possibility of Comprehensive education. The local Church of England Comprehensive has a special unit for the physically handicapped. There is a great deal of integration into the rest of the school, but it provides a sheltered base for those who need it. We hope Lizzie will be able to attend that school when the time comes.

We know we will have to wait until Lizzie reaches her last year at the primary school before deciding. Whatever happens, we would like to pursue the possibility of continued integration. Lizzie is still within the range of the ability of the class she is in. If she continues to progress in this way, and we have no evidence to suggest she won't, we are hopeful.

If it becomes clear that she would not be happy at a Comprehensive, we may perhaps consider something else. But until she tries, we won't know, and neither will she.

9

Lizzie and Family Life

'Can you think of something funny Lizzie did?' I asked Nick.
'I think the funniest thing was when we went shopping. Do you remember? That trolley..!'

We drove along the straight road to Asda, over the canal, under the railway bridge with musical notes painted across it and then down to the traffic lights. A tape of music was being accompanied by Lizzie's gruff tones. Susie was in the baby seat. Nick sat next to her, looking out of the window.

I indicated right, drew over into the centre of the road and then we were driving into the huge car park entrance and scanning the parking lots for a space.

The tarmac was black with rain and as we got out of the car, I grabbed Susie's hand to stop her crossing the roadway, and told Lizzie to hold onto Nick.

We entered the green-and-white store, a box of delights for young eyes, and found a trolley. There were arguments about who should ride in it, but Susannah won. We were inside. I clutched my list—and my stomach suddenly lurched. It was a throw-back to the past, when entering a supermarket had always been a source of anxiety. I reminded myself that it would be all right now: Lizzie was much more sensible. Shopping was not the nightmare it had once been. Gone were the days when she would run off and it would take me ten minutes of precious time to find her, time for babies to get hungry, time for toddlers to get fractious. There had been quite a long period when I simply would not take all three children shopping. I felt too awful at the end of it. It wasn't worth it. I'd resort to going alone after tea, between 6 and 7 p.m., while Mark bathed them.

But we had progressed. Shopping was usually more peaceful these days, apart from some inter-sibling rivalry and frequent requests for crisps.

Today I noticed some price-reduced children's wear and I pushed the trolley towards the racks. Lizzie needed some new jeans. I was glad to see they had some in her size. I let go of the trolley to compare styles. I felt pleased we could now afford to buy her some new clothes and not be so dependent on sources of secondhand ones. It was nice to feel she could look modern. She loved wearing trousers. There were two kinds of jeans—which ones would be best? I turned to Lizzie to see which she would like. Lizzie wasn't there, nor was the trolley.

'Oh no,' I thought. My heart sank. I had visions of her collecting and eating boxes of chocolates—like the day she had run off to the Easter egg stand and returned a few minutes later, half of one huge Easter egg eaten, the rest in torn foil. Thankfully the assistants were understanding, but I had felt very embarrassed.

I suggested Nick might walk round one set of aisles while I walked round some others. He returned moments later, no sign of Lizzie. I held the chosen jeans and we walked along the yoghurt section, past the biscuit aisle, past the jams and puddings, to the vegetables.

Time was passing. Where on earth was Lizzie and what was she doing? We walked down other unusually empty aisles. No Lizzie in sight. I was really getting worried now. Whatever she had done was bound to be time-consuming to put right.

And then we saw her. A small girl in sweatshirt and trousers, pushing a huge trolley half-full of food along the soft drinks section. She reached for some lemonade. Grandpa always had lemonade for the children when we visited.

We came up behind Lizzie. 'We don't want any of these, Lizzie, what have you been doing?' I said anxiously. Then I

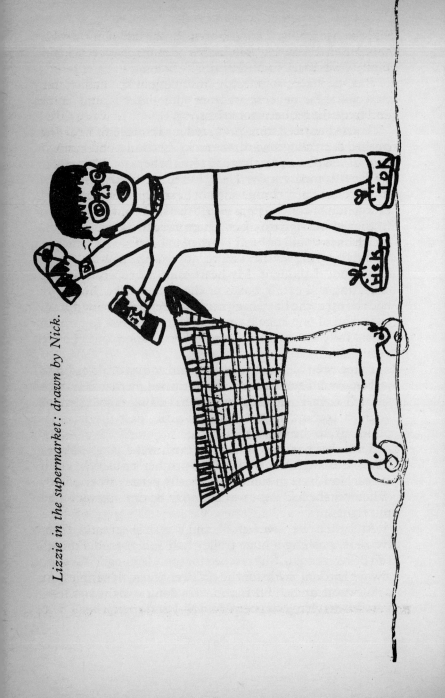

Lizzie in the supermarket: drawn by Nick.

looked in her trolley. I was amazed. It was full of our weekly shop. Granted, she had put in two or more of everything—but there was the yoghurt I normally bought, the margarine, the cheese, the biscuits. She explained that she had chosen some processed cheese because she liked it and some chocolate biscuits because she liked them too—'was it OK?'

We all laughed with relief. Lizzie had come of age. She knew what to buy. She was very sensible and observant, I realized. I suddenly felt proud of her.

We gently put back a large number of bottles of Schweppes bitter lemon, and congratulated Lizzie on her choices. I needn't worry about shopping, I decided as we walked to the check-out. Perhaps I could even send Lizzie instead? Well, perhaps not!

I used to be encumbered with huge bags of nappies after a big shop—but not now. That was another area where Lizzie had suddenly grown up. I could hardly believe we had only begun to potty train her at night this summer. It seemed years ago.

Training

As we drove home, I absently wondered if we had tried to potty train her far too early in the first place. Perhaps that was why it had been so hard. But she couldn't have gone to nursery school if she hadn't been in pants.

We certainly hadn't pushed her too hard about night times. Rather than wash sheets every night, I decided to wait until she woke up with a dry nappy before I let her sleep without one. The problem was that she passed her eighth birthday and still never woke with a dry nappy. The consultant told us that unless we left her nappy off, she would never be dry. But how could I wash sheets and duvet covers—duvets even—every day? I had so many other things to do.

So we ignored his statement and went on with nappies. At least it was painless. Then came the historic night at school camp, when Lizzie had been dry, with her teacher's help. The truth slowly dawned. I would have to do what the headmistress had done and wake myself up if we were ever going to help her. If we could discover when she needed to go to the loo, and gradually bring the time nearer to when we went to bed, we might win. I decided to take the plunge and set my alarm for 3 a.m. I volunteered first. Mark could do it when I had had enough.

A bell rang in the middle of a deep and peaceful sleep. What on earth was happening? I grabbed for the alarm. What a horrible noise. Feeling slightly sick, I realized what I was supposed to be doing, got up and put Lizzie on the loo. Success. Then I got back under the warm duvet and tried to sleep.

It was hopeless. I tossed and turned until 4 a.m. before I drifted off. Next day I wondered how I'd cope with the lack of sleep if this went on for months. I could see why waking prisoners up at 3 a.m. was a well-known form of torture.

Why did it feel so different from getting up to feed a tiny baby? Sleep had never been slow in coming then.

The next night I woke before the alarm and waited for its raucous noise, then realized I could simply turn it off.

I was grumpy and short-tempered all day. It was no good. I'd be a nervous wreck before this was over. On the third morning, despite our actions, Lizzie's bed was wet. Could Mark get up instead? He doesn't sleep very well anyway.

But the next night Lizzie woke us 1 a.m. to say she had wet the bed. So we decided to set the alarm for earlier. Next night we tried two o'clock. It worked. Gradually, over the next few days, we brought it forward by half an hour... Until, after three weeks, we were waking at midnight and Lizzie was dry more often than not.

A few more weeks and we were able to take her to the toilet when we went to bed. The transformation was complete. At first there were a few accidents, but not many. Then there were none.

I wondered again, as I drove the car home, if the fact that Lizzie was dry at night and had also learned to swim (with the help of armbands) had any relation to the time of special prayer for her when we were on holiday. Since then I had made a special point of offering Lizzie to God each night as she went to sleep. Whatever the reason, I was grateful for the progress. These were major steps for Lizzie in growing up and gaining her own independence.

Behaviour can change

Lizzie's self-esteem has improved since she has stopped wearing nappies. She is very quick to point out that she doesn't wear nappies any more if there is a baby around. Her attitudes to clothes and her appearance have changed too. She is more willing these days to discuss what colours go together and what makes her look pretty.

We have resorted to a number of incentives to improve Lizzie's behaviour this year. Refusing to wipe her nose, or get dressed in the morning, or to help tidy her clothes, were things that annoyed me. One day we suddenly discovered that Lizzie blew her own nose at school... So who was she kidding! I made a sticker chart. Now I have a queue of helpful children wanting to lay the table, make sandwiches, tidy rooms—to get stickers, because there is a surprise present when there are twenty stickers on the chart! Nowadays Lizzie always wipes her own nose and usually gets dressed on her own. She is noticeably more helpful.

A psychology book that I remember more for its title than its contents is called *Behaviour Can Change*. It is good to be reminded of that when the going gets tough!

Games

Lizzie and Susie seem to get on better now than they used to. Lizzie at nine and Susie at four have discovered the power of being allies—two strong-minded girls who sometimes plot to exclude their brother. Yet both adore Nick and their feuds don't last long. They play many pretend games together, especially schools, where Richard, Lizzie's school friend, is always Lizzie's naughty pupil.

'Bands' is another favourite game. Mum and Dad reluctantly sit on the hall carpet while Lizzie stands importantly at the bottom of the stairs. Nick comes from upstairs, sunglasses on and wearing a denim jacket, miming a guitar.

Lizzie announces proudly: 'A big hand for...' (the latest pop singer). Susannah emerges sheepishly and we clap. Lizzie gets the timing of her announcement just right and she laughs with delight.

We then receive the latest version of a Jason Donovan song...with Philps additions. Sometimes there are paper guitars and microphones made from string and pens attached to the loud speakers of our music centre.

'Meetings' is usually a game Lizzie plays on her own: books and pens are placed on each chair in the sitting-room. The first time she played this game was in the old big vicarage. There I emerged from the bedroom one morning to find the enormous bare-boarded landing covered in Mark's scrap paper, a pencil neatly placed beside each piece of paper, with a doll or animal next to it. She had learnt how to match one to one, if nothing else.

Some of Lizzie's games have been taken up by the other two. They all like having desks and writing at them. Perhaps this is also because Mum and Dad spend a lot of their time writing at desks, too! Lizzie likes writing more than any other game. It used to annoy me, because Lizzie seemed always to write rubbish. She simply wanted to cover a page. She refused to copy from a book or words I'd write for her. Then someone told me about 'emergent' writing, and one day I realized that perhaps I'd be able to understand some of the words on the page.

Nowadays Lizzie will write pretend letters to people, and a few of the words are quite correct. Her current obsession is 'joined-up writing', and she produces long pages of beautiful writing patterns!

Sometimes I have felt she is obsessed by the outward appearance of things without understanding the contents.

But my impatience has often been confounded. The contents do come eventually and they are worth waiting for.

Brother and sister
You often hear stories of the siblings of handicapped people being left to look after them, making their own lives miserably frustrating.

I hope all three of our children have their own place in the family. Now that Lizzie is more independent, it is certainly easier. Nick loves books, and I have found that when we choose bedtime books with Nick in mind, Lizzie is quite happy to listen. She listens to Susie's book too, which I secretly feel she enjoys more. But Lizzie also has her own 'special time' when we do spelling games or a computer programme and work through her reading book. Sometimes Daddy plays chess with Nick, or makes a model, while this is happening.

There are occasions when Nick might enjoy something that Lizzie wouldn't, but they are becoming fewer. Nick goes to Beavers on his own and Lizzie to her beloved 714 Club at church. As they grow and develop their own interests, it becomes easier for them to express their individuality.

Car journeys can become a time of tension. Lizzie's hearing is not perfect and she often asks for the volume of the tape to be turned up and is grumpy when it isn't. She also tends to muscle her way in to television watching and tends to sit in front of the screen if she isn't firmly prevented from doing so.

But perhaps our family's love of books has rubbed off on Lizzie too. She had taken a paperback to 'read' on one car journey. It was much too difficult, but I heard her 'reading' aloud. She described 'the sea so blue...the wind blowing...' and used many descriptive phrases. I wished I could have recorded it on tape. On another journey she looked out at the winter landscape and said, 'I see trees and the distant hills', and announced that she was going to remember it 'in her brain' and draw it when we got home—which she did. She drew a picture of wintery trees without leaves on a hill.

She makes up her own songs on her toy guitar. 'I just want to know you are there or not.' She sounded very professional as she strummed the guitar. I think she was referring to God.

Her imagination is full of jokes. One day she decided she had an imaginary friend called St Nicholas who was handicapped and had to go in a wheelchair (pronounced 'wheelen chair'). In the bath she talked about 'Jumbo the 16th coming tomorrow'. We were looking after a baby the following day.

Lizzie's jokes are improving as she grows up. The 'knock knock, who's there' variety are the best at the moment.

Co-operation

Lizzie finds it hard to deceive anyone. She will approach me grinning wildly, showing me empty hands, and I can guarantee she has something she shouldn't have in her pocket.

The worst situations are in a shopping centres, when she takes something from one shop and gives it to me in another. I feel like a criminal as we take it back. Thankfully we don't all go shopping often!

Going to the loo, and washing hands before tea, are opportunities for deception. 'I went yesterday' she will say seriously. We all burst out laughing. Then she'll say 'yes' to questions about hand washing but her grin tells us otherwise.

It is not hard to find out the truth.

Lizzie is much happier these days. But those ignorant people who dare to say, 'all Down's people are so happy aren't they?' get a quizzical glare from me.

During Lizzie's first three years at full-time school, the new demands made upon her and her smallness of stature produced tiredness, grumpiness and unkind, aggressive, possessive behaviour. Only in retrospect can I see that she has grown out of this gradually over the last year, and is much more equable and pleasant. She is more co-operative and

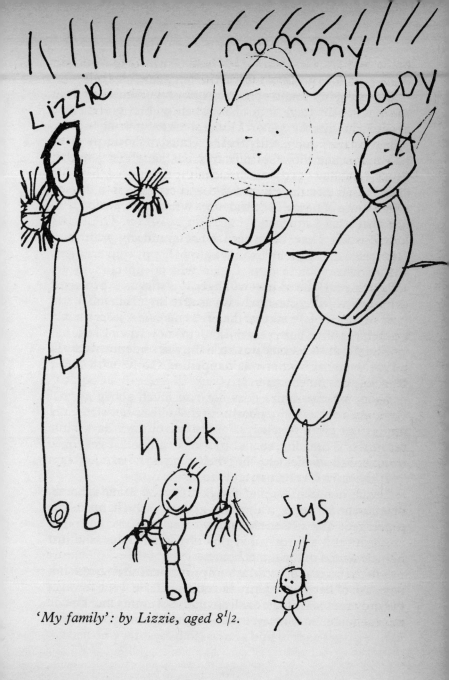

'My family': by Lizzie, aged 8¹/2.

polite, and kinder to Susie and Nick. She is more willing to share treasured possessions like her felt pens.

Psychologists would perhaps speak of the transition from the egocentric stage into one of being able to see other people's points of view. Mothers often talk about the struggles they have with their exhausted, grumpy five-year-olds when they return from school, and the calm that gradually follows as they get used to the rigours of school life and emerge into the six-year-old and seven-year-old stage with a sense of peaceful confidence. Whatever we call it, I'm just glad it has happened.

In the past, I have often been so fed up and angry with her. It is a relief now to be able to have lots of happy conversations and cuddles. These days Lizzie will go upstairs to get something for one of us—willingly if a sticker is promised as a reward—whereas she always used to say, 'I am too tired.'

It's at times of illness that the tired bolshiness rears its ugly head. It has often been very difficult to know when Lizzie has been really ill. When she was little she was sometimes very ill before I realized what was happening. Now, with fewer illnesses, it is much easier.

Lizzie's temperature does not rise much above normal even when she is quite poorly, so if she feels hot she really needs to be taken seriously. For the two or three days while the illness is brewing, she is often very difficult. I get angry with her and wonder why she is behaving as she is. A few days later she has a sore throat, and the penny drops.

She is a good actress, and if Nick or Susie is ill and at home, there may be tears when she gets up which make me concerned. Then I see her empty cereal bowl at the end of breakfast and am reassured that she is all right. She just wanted to join in the fun at home.

Another area of gradual improvement has been her response to babysitting arrangements. Lizzie went through a phase of refusing to go to sleep unless Mummy and Daddy were at home. So whenever we went out for a meal, or to see a film, we'd get back to find a harassed babysitter who had got

Lizzie to sleep only ten minutes before, after hours of cajoling, or reading stories until she was hoarse.

Lizzie was very grumpy the following day, because she was so overtired, and we really wondered if it was worth going out. We seemed to pay a lot for it, one way or another.

Gradually Lizzie began to accept babysitters. And now there are several she will actually go to sleep for. She needed to build up trust in a situation that was strange and probably far more confusing for Lizzie than for us.

One of the family

At my parents' Ruby Wedding anniversary party, Lizzie appeared with a scarf and a box before an audience of relatives and friends. 'Abracadabra' she announced, very loudly, and whipped the scarf away to reveal the box. When she tried to make the box disappear it didn't work quite as well, but it was all good fun.

Lizzie loves drama. I hope that one day she will be able to join a drama group, or take part in our church drama group. She certainly enjoys acting at home.

Drama on television is a hot favourite: Narnia stories, classic dramas, even soap operas if we allowed them, all keep Lizzie happy. We have to ration the television, so that there is time to play with Susie and Nick, which helps her development more. Yet sometimes seeing a film has stimulated Lizzie's enjoyment of a story and helped her understand the book.

Lizzie has a strong sense of belonging to our family. This became very clear when she decided, after a couple of sessions at her disco dancing class, that she wanted to be 'altogether' on Saturdays. She refused to go any more. Saturday is the day we try to keep for doing things together as a family, and Lizzie did not want to miss out.

As a family, we value meal times too, when we are all seated around the kitchen table. Lizzie's conversations are currently punctuated by questions about 'ingredients'. This may have been started by a school cookery lesson, but any food placed on the table is put through the ritual. It has to be analysed, and if the list of ingredients is not long enough and Lizzie repeats the question 'But what are its 'gredients?' it is not unknown for a desperate parent to invent a few.

Thumps on the table sometimes greet the arrival of an unwelcome dish, but on the whole Lizzie has extended her range of 'acceptable' meals since infancy. This is a great relief, since her staple diet as a toddler was bananas and minced meat stew. Bananas are less popular now than peanut-butter sandwiches, and if Lizzie was to be marooned on a desert island, peanut-butter sandwiches would be essential to her survival.

10
Lizzie and Church

*Jesus said: 'Unless you become like little
children, you will never enter the
Kingdom of heaven.'*

It was lunch-time. I walked down the deserted passageway
towards the large theatre where the children's activities were
being held for the week. I had ten minutes before the children
surged out of the doors, a huge mass of talking, happy,
hungry youngsters. They would be bursting to share the
excitements of the morning, the songs they had sung, the
stories that had been told.

I savoured the last silent moments. The sound of singing
drifted towards me from across the passage. I peered through
a porthole window in the green door and saw people sitting
facing an overhead projector. Someone was playing a guitar. I
gently pushed the door open and slid inside, hoping no one
would notice me. As I stood at the back of the room, people
began to get up and walk around. They were clutching pieces
of red paper which I realized were heart-shaped.

'Take your heart and give it to someone else in the room. As
you give them your heart you are telling them you love them.
You are sharing God's love.'

I watched as people slowly rose from their seats and moved
towards each other. Suddenly I felt tears running down my
face. Why did this scene move me so much? The room was
full of mentally handicapped young adults. This was the
special seminar at Spring Harvest, a Christian holiday and

teaching week held at several Butlins centres each Easter. I had never been to such a meeting before. There was great warmth and reality in the simple worship.

Lizzie's own faith has gone through different phases. Lizzie has always encouraged me to pray for people, and asks for a prayer when she goes to sleep. She reminds us if we have forgotten to say grace before meals, or the family Bible story we read at supper time. But now Lizzie is beginning to think things out for herself. She finds it hard, for example, to understand that God can be with us if he is also in heaven.

She enjoys and remembers the Bible stories she hears at home, school and Sunday school. She remembers the wise man who built his house on the rock, and Samson who was very strong. She loves the Christian music tapes we play in the car. Sometimes, being slightly deaf, she has threatened us in the car with, 'If you don't turn the tape up, I'll stop singing.' We laugh, as Lizzie's singing is often rather gruff and very loud. It is becoming more tuneful, but a tape and Lizzie singing on a journey can be a bit much.

At our church Lizzie likes to sit in the same pew every week with the other Sunday School children. She complains and shunts every one around if someone else has taken her place. She feels happier with a familiar routine.

She loves to sit and watch and join in the singing. She is keen to have a hymn book open at the right hymn, and she often sneaks one out, to carry on with the service at home afterwards.

It's a special treat for Lizzie to go to the evening service. This we do occasionally for events like the Christmas carol service. This year I took part in some dance drama and afterwards Lizzie said how much she liked watching me. She loves our band, the drums, guitar and keyboard which help lead the worship. For Lizzie, church is a happy place. She belongs.

Whenever we visit a new town and happen to go inside the church, Lizzie will collect a prayer book and start to conduct a service from the altar steps. Church is home to her.

One Sunday morning we got there early. There was no one there except Mark, sorting out his materials and the overhead projector sheets.

I wandered slowly up the blue-carpeted aisle, looking at the simple wooden altar panels and the warm red and white of the chancel roof. Lizzie had just reached the communion table. She had collected a glass of water from Mark's pew and stood near the table facing the front. She dipped her fingers into the water and then touched her forehead with it.

'What are you doing, Lizzie?' I asked. 'I'm making the Down's Syndrome go away, Mummy. I don't want it any more. I'm baptising myself, like Daddy does.'

Perhaps Lizzie had confused prayer for healing with baptism, but she took it all very seriously.

At home, her games reflect the activities of her parents. So the chairs are put out in the sitting-room at 7 a.m., with a pencil, a sheet of paper and a song book on every seat. 'A meeting,' says Lizzie. She will then proceed to conduct her own meeting, which may be a Bible study or Sunday School. The latter always has her friend Richard as the naughty boy. Her deep voice penetrates the floorboards into our bedroom above. 'You really are very naughty today, Richard.'

714 Club, our church's club for children aged seven to fourteen, is the high spot of Lizzie's week. It is the first club she has gone to alone. In the church hall, with friends from school and the neighbourhood, Lizzie plays snooker, football, and paints. She joins in the simple Bible quiz or story time at the end, and returns at 8 p.m. full of beans.

It is noisy, but she loves it. The 714 Disco was much talked about and looked forward to. Lizzie decided she wouldn't wear her black skirt, which I thought looked very smart. She explained the reason in a very grown-up fashion. 'I'll wear a T-shirt under my tracksuit, so that if I get hot I can take off the top.' I didn't have the heart to insist on my choice. I left her dancing with the others in the hall, suddenly feeling that she had grown up. Certainly she has grown up a lot since our arrival here. When we first came there were times when

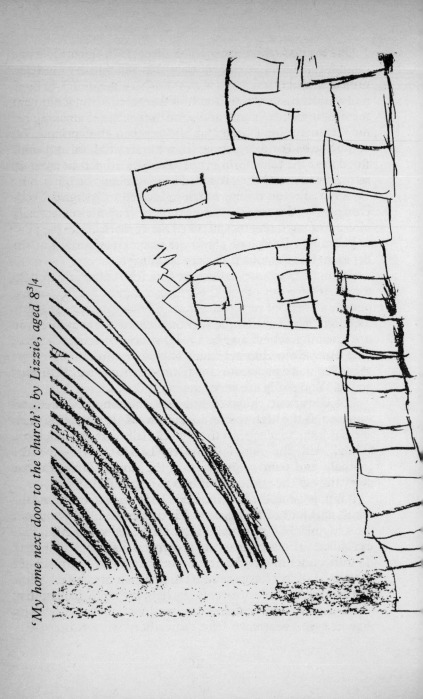

'My home next door to the church': by Lizzie, aged 8¾

Lizzie would lie on the carpet in the aisle in the middle of a church service and everyone would have to walk round her. Or she would refuse to go with the others to Sunday School, and sit at the back of the church on the table, writing. Now she joins in—keen to be part of the life of the church, making her own contribution of quiet faithfulness and absorption.

When the children return from Sunday School and come forward to the Communion rail to be blessed, Lizzie roars up to the front at a fast walk, proud to kneel and be blessed by Daddy. She feels very much at home and slightly self-conscious. She gives a sideways grin but doesn't actually look at me until afterwards, when she comes back to the pew. She sometimes likes to stand next to me and sing, but she often prefers to be with the other children.

Some people have developed a special relationship with Lizzie. Those who know her well would probably agree that she gives a kind of acceptance that does not threaten. She does not make demands. She is not someone who is weighing you up, to see whether or not you have got it right. Because of that, a relationship with Lizzie can bring its own healing for those who may feel hurt and let down by others and unable to trust many people with their real feelings.

So much could be done to make handicapped children and adults truly welcome in churches. Many families with handicapped members are very isolated. Belonging to a church community could dissolve that isolation. And in the process everyone could gain from the contribution the handicapped person can make to the church.

Ability is not a prerequisite for learning about the Christian faith. Sharing our lives, our problems and our joys, is part of life in a church family. It is something we can all contribute to at any level. The church could help, too, in caring for those trying to come to terms with the birth of a handicapped child, or to cope with the isolation felt when the child is bussed to school some miles away, or the isolation of being housebound because you are looking after a severely handicapped person.

Jean Vanier is the founder of the L'Arche communities. These communities—now in several countries—are places where the handicapped and able-bodied live on equal terms. These moving words come from his book, *The Broken Body*:

'Perhaps we can be a sign of the value of each person, no matter how broken, no matter how poor or how apparently useless he or she may appear to society. A sign that they carry a treasure in their hearts.

'Perhaps through our struggle to save and help one person to find freedom we are struggling for all humanity and all the oppressed.

'Perhaps we can help reveal the secret of the Gospels: that God chooses what is foolish in order to confound the wise; that God chooses what is weak in order to confound the strong; that God chooses what is lowest and most despised to reveal his power and glory.

'Thus we can help to call forth others to walk on the downward path, the path of humility and compassion, so that people may discover for themselves the saving power of the Gospels: Jesus, the Lamb, who comes to bring peace to the world by taking away sin and opening our hearts to the poor and the broken, so that together we can celebrate our oneness and grow to freedom. For the glory of God in the wholeness of his Body is each human person fully alive.'

Perhaps the specialness of that Spring Harvest seminar was not that the individuals were handicapped but that other people were at last taking them seriously. Their own simple expression of faith was valued for what it truly was: an act of worship of great value to the God who created them.

11
Lizzie and Holidays

'What is the favourite thing you like about holidays, Lizzie?' I asked.

'A bonfire on the beach and camping at Granny's,' she replied.

We drove down the now familiar factory-lined street to the dual carriageway and turned left. We were going south—down the M5, then off to the left again along roads becoming familiar with more frequent use. Roundabouts, restaurants, hedges, fields, trees and then the chalklands—where I spent my first year teaching, the year we got engaged and then married. Dry, treeless, smoothly rounded hills, distinctive, unique. We were near our destination: the home of friends who lived in a beautiful small country town. We'd arrived. The children piled out of the car, glad to move and breathe freely again. Even Narnia tapes hadn't enthralled them for the whole journey. There is a limit to a child's endurance of confinement.

There is excitement in their voices as we walk down the drive to the house. Is Edward there? Yes! Lizzie runs to meet him. Two short, stocky children walk hand in hand. Their gait is similar. They both wear glasses. But there the similarities end. Edward has Down's Syndrome too. He is the same age as Lizzie. They look sufficiently alike for someone to mistake Lizzie for Edward in the town on a shopping trip. But their personalities establish their individuality.

Edward is quiet and peaceful; Lizzie is often noisy and

temperamental. Edward is not aggressive; Lizzie often winds people up, then kicks and pushes them if they react badly. Lizzie has to be restrained from running Edward's life for him when she goes to stay. He is well capable of making his own decisions but Lizzie wants to mother him and organize him, as others have organized her. Edward is sensitive to the heavy control and complains to his Mum. Edward is obedient and gentle; Lizzie is disobedient and rough. But they like each other.

We parents get annoyed that people often lump Down's children together. We can testify that they are far more like themselves, far more like their families, than they are like each other. Outward appearances are deceptive.

We walk down to the adventure playground, wood chips crunching under foot. I notice that the children play more independently than they did the last time we came. The river bends round the playground. Low-rise flats, their bay windows protruding out over the water, follow the line of the river.

I stand and stare. The contrast with home engulfs me. For a moment I am homesick for other places and other times. But I know now that I must turn away from self-pity. God brings us to the places he chooses, and if we are where he wants he will bless us. Our circumstances do not determine our inner joy and fulfilment.

Holidays are important times for taking stock of our lives and lifestyles—seeing them through different eyes. We are always stimulated and refreshed as we drive back to the Midlands after a few days' break.

Holidays can sometimes be a problem for clergy. Money will not stretch to hotels or, usually, to visits abroad, yet we need to spend time out of the parish to have a break.

Lizzie thrives on routine, partly because it is hard for her mind to grasp new things. Holidays can be difficult for her. That holiday in Paris when Lizzie was young had highlighted the problem for us. A week nearer home, in the Peak District, underlined it again.

We were in our trailer tent. Lizzie was not yet able to go to bed without a nappy and I had not discovered that the clinic would provide us with larger, child-sized nappies free of charge.

It was 1.30 a.m. and raining when Lizzie woke up. Perhaps she had eaten something that had upset her. The nappy had leaked, all over the sleeping-bag, the bed and the tent wall.

I dragged myself out of bed and followed Mark to the stove. We fumbled around for matches, a kettle and water. I was in a state of mild panic. How on earth could we sort all this out on holiday in a tent? It was bad enough at home. I was crying by now and angry with Lizzie. It was one of those desperate moments. But we sorted things out in the end—you have to!

The Peak district is lovely if you like walking. But Lizzie didn't. She couldn't see the point unless she was distracted by eating something or playing a game. Mark's shoulders and my back ached from carrying our solid seven-year-old.

We thought disloyally of how Nick and Susie managed it all so easily and enjoyed the scenery. Secretly we fumed. It would be easier without Lizzie on this holiday. Guiltily we plotted to send her to grandparents for the week—but we knew we never would. That would be conceding defeat.

Or would it? Was it defeat or realism? Were we too hooked on making Lizzie 'normal' regardless? Shouldn't we sometimes make some allowances?

Last summer the sun shone and shone. England in the sun is far more beautiful in my eyes than anywhere else. We spent every day on the beach, surfing, digging castles. By now we had graduated from the tent to a more home-like caravan.

Lizzie had progressed beyond the awful stage she was in a few years ago, when every family on the beach was more interesting than her own. She would plonk herself on her victims' beach mat and ask for a share in their lunch. She often got it, too. But I was embarrassed. I was always tracking her round the beach, rescuing her from unsuspecting victims.

Now she stayed nearer to our belongings, aped the sun-worshippers by sprawling on a mat, looking at a book. Occasionally she watched other children build castles; and even more occasionally she dug one herself. But the sea did not attract her and she rarely went near it.

Beach holidays, when the weather is good, are exactly what Lizzie likes. If Lizzie is happy, so are we. But if Lizzie is difficult about something that doesn't mean we won't do it. I don't want us to feel we are missing out through having Lizzie. I've sometimes had to encourage Mark to persevere with a visit to some National Trust property (which he enjoys), because memories of having to carry Lizzie round to prevent her from touching everything still linger. Now, Lizzie looks at everything with interest and announces that each four-poster bed she sees was slept in by King Charles. These days, though, we are less ambitious than we once were—or more realistic.

Swimming has always been something Lizzie has found difficult. She loved to float around the warm hydrotherapy pool as a baby, and at eighteen months would swim on her own with armbands. I thought I had a genius on my hands. But when Nick was on the way, and we were some distance from any warm pool, we stopped swimming regularly.

When I was able to take both the children, Lizzie was frightened and wouldn't come in the water at all. She would sit on the side with her feet dangling, getting cold.

We discovered a swimming-pool with a wave machine and graded edges, and spent a whole week of Mark's holiday in and out of the pool when Nick was still in his carry cot on the side. Lizzie began to go into the water again. Gradually, through persistent visits, she began to walk in the shallow area and lie down and splash. We had to be very patient and she often refused to wear armbands. Despite lessons at school and weekly visits to the pool, she would sit on the side or splash in the shallow end. Every time I said, 'Shall I help you swim, Lizzie?', an adamant 'No' was the response.

It wasn't until the summer when she was eight that she

swam a few strokes on her own, wearing armbands. It began when she discovered she could float on her bottom, kicking her legs, sitting up in the water. Then she tried swimming on her front and, to her delight as well as ours, she could do it. Like other things, it seems that she had waited until she had perfected the art in her mind, then she had done it. But that did not detract from her triumph that day—and, rewarded by crisps and a promise of how pleased Daddy would be, we drove home.

Our experience with swimming underlined for me Lizzie's sensitivity and her fear of the unknown. We are fortunate to have a lovely warm learner pool at our local baths—I hope this year she will learn to swim properly.

New environments do pose problems. We have left the children for a night just twice so far, once with my parents and once with my sister. Lizzie demonstrated her anxiety by wetting the bed four times in a hour on the latter occasion! Somehow this revealed for me the utter stupidity of the statement made the night after Lizzie was born: 'Oh, they don't know who brings them up!' Lizzie's attachment to me is no different from that of my other children.

The safety and security of routine, and therefore the problems holidays might bring, was underlined for me once by a friend with an autistic child. It really helped him to sleep in the same room every year when he went on a holiday held in a large, confusing, school building. We have decided that at present it is more relaxing for all of us if we go to the same place each year and Lizzie always has the same bed in the caravan!

Our parish weekend was held on a farm in Shropshire. It was the second year we had stayed there, so Lizzie was familiar with the place. When we arrived, the children rushed up the metal staircase to their room overlooking the concrete football area which was once the farmyard and into the bedroom area. 'Same room as last year?' asked Nick. 'No,' I said, as I showed them into a room on their own. They had shared ours last year. The children started to unpack their clothes and put them in the drawers. 'Our own wash basin,' said Lizzie. Mark and I threw our things into the room next door and we went downstairs to sort out the food.

On the following morning I awoke at 6 a.m. Something had disturbed me. I crept out of bed and pushed open the door to the children's room. Lizzie wasn't there, but the outside door of the building was locked. I was puzzled, but feeling too lazy to get up properly I went back to bed, firmly pulling up the sheet and snuggling down. I told myself she must be in with our friends who were sleeping across the corridor.

At seven o'clock I decided I ought to find out what was happening. I heard my friend come out of her room and I asked her if she had Lizzie. 'No,' she said.

I unlocked the front door and stared across the farmyard. Lizzie was emerging from the large conference room, clutching a Bible. I called out to ask her what she was doing? 'Having my prayer time and reading my Bible' she replied indignantly. 'How could you be so silly as not to realize,' she implied.

How had she got out, I wondered?

As I went back into the children's bedroom I noticed the curtain flapping. The window was wide open!

12
Family Relationships

I am often asked what effect Lizzie has on family relationships. How do her brother and sister feel? How does Mark feel? And what kind of stress does a handicapped child put on a marriage?

When Nick was six and Lizzie was eight and three-quarters I recorded the following conversation. The questions are mine: the answers are Nick's.

Can you say what it feels like to have Lizzie as your sister?
If I didn't have her in my family it wouldn't be the same.

What is special about her for you?
I like the games she plays. She's kind to me.

Do you ever feel sad that she has Down's Syndrome?
Yes I do, quite a lot of the time.

Why do you feel sad?
Because I feel sorry for her.

Why do you feel sorry? Because she can't do as much as you?
Yes.

Do you think you've learnt anything good from it?
I might be someone when I'm older who looks after people with Down's Syndrome, and it helps me learn how to do that.

Do you think Mummy and Daddy spend more time with Lizzie than you?
Sometimes.

Often?
Not often.

At school, do you think people pay more attention to Lizzie than you?
No, not at school.

What do you like doing best with Lizzie?
Getting up in the morning and playing 'schools' with her.

Do you like doing things with Mummy and Daddy on your own?
I like it very much, like reading stories.

Do you feel you have enough time with them on your own?
Not when guests come, but normally it is all right.

What is the funniest thing Lizzie has ever done?
Dressing up as a clown with face paints, playing bands.

Then I questioned Lizzie.

Can you describe yourself Lizzie? Are you happy or sad? Kind or unkind? Bossy, or do you like looking after people?
I am kind and helpful. I am happy. Sometimes I be unhappy because Nick is hurting me.

Do you think you are bossy?
No.

Do you like telling other people what to do?
No. Well, yes—Richard.

At school?
Yes.

Do you think everyone likes you?
Yes, in my class.

So you have lots of friends?
Yes.

Are you tall or short, Lizzie?
Tall.

Lizzie is my sister.

the best thing about
her is she like's
playing the same
thing's as me.
Like handeekapt
Sch*ool's. I staeted
the game of.
the thiny I don't
Like about her is
that she anhoys
me. I wothned like
are family with out Lizzie
in it. I Like seeiny
her in the playground
at fhool by Nick Aage 1
6 4

Thin or fat?
Thin.

Pretty or ugly?
Pretty... (Then Lizzie got worried. 'You said I was ugly.'
Rapid explanations were needed before she was reassured.)

Peaceful or do you get worried?
No, I don't worry. I like having a fire to keep warm at. (A
reference to weekend 'crash outs' in the winter, when we play
games around a wood fire. This is popular with all the family.)

Are you very busy in the day?
Yes, sometimes. Not always.

Are you good at dancing, or bad?
Good. (She said the same about reading, sums and writing.)

Are you well behaved?
Sometimes.

Do you get told off? For talking?
Sometimes. To be quiet, to be in silence, do work in silence. I
don't want to work in silence.

What do you want to do?
Talk to Richard.

Do you think Mummy loves you?
Yes.

Daddy?
No, because he keeps shouting at me.

Do you love Daddy?
No.

Why?
I just don't.

Poor Daddy, do you think he would be sad if he knew?
I do really. I'm just joking. I love everyone in my family. I
know what I am in my family. That means good. I am good.

Do you think God and Jesus love you?
Yes.

Are they pleased with you?
Yes.

Is that a nice feeling?
Yes. I like Miss Hall too.

Is she pleased with you?
Yes, sometimes.

Usually? When is she cross with you?
When eat in silence.

You mean in the dining room? Do you throw food?
My children in my class do. I don't, and Richard doesn't.
(This may not be quite true!)

One last question Lizzie. Do you think you are good at drawing?
Yes.

What do you think you are best at?
Drawing, dancing and writing.

Thank you, Lizzie. That was very good.

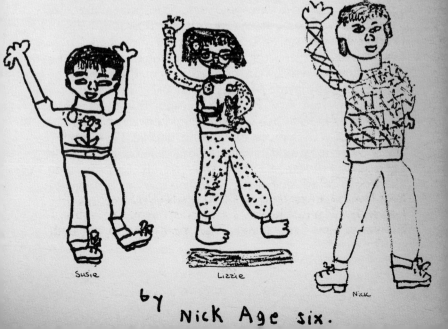

Susie   Lizzie   Nick

by Nick Age six.

A father's view

My memory of Elizabeth coming into this world is vivid: she shot into the bright light of the labour ward as if catapulted or fired from a popgun. The midwife, urging Caroline to push hard, had naturally not reckoned on Lizzie weighing only 4lbs—hence the uncontrolled arrival.

What happened afterwards is equally vivid. There was an immediate change in the atmosphere. Not the joyful recognition of the presence of another human being which normally accompanies even the toughest delivery, but an emptiness, a flatness, a sense of anti-climax. Hardly a word was spoken. Lizzie was wrapped up and a doctor called in to examine her. Then she was whisked away to be put in an incubator, with a muttered explanation that her temperature was low.

Some time later I was called to the special baby-care unit to see her. The nurse took the bundle out of the incubator and put it into my arms. I did what I imagined good fathers were supposed to do and cuddled her as gently as I could, sitting nervously on the edge of a chair. Again little was said. And after a few minutes, feeling slightly foolish, I called for the nurse and handed the bundle back.

Looking back, I can of course interpret what was happening with some assurance. The medical staff realized immediately they saw, and more particularly touched, Lizzie that something was wrong; and it cannot have been long before they had a shrewd idea what the something was. The reason for calling me to the special baby-care unit was probably twofold: first, knowing that something was wrong they wanted to establish a relationship between parent and child, to begin the process of bonding, hoping that when the bad news came I would have gone too far in knowing Lizzie as a person to be able to reject her. And secondly, I imagine they wanted me to ask questions, to realize that something was wrong, or might be wrong, and to give them the opening they needed in order to talk.

I have never been quick on the uptake and I was

particularly slow then. At some level I sensed that all was not as it should be, but that realization never came quite near enough to consciousness for me to lay hold of it and express it. So I felt foolish, sitting around with Lizzie in my arms in the special baby-care unit because I knew that in some way I had failed, I had not responded to the unexpressed hopes of the staff.

I should have known better. Part of the mercy of God in the situation was that I had worked with handicapped children, including a number of Down's children, before.

After leaving school I had most of a year to make some use of before going to university. I spent some months pursuing lost causes and wildly inappropriate ideas, from a half-baked plan to go to Nepal and tend to the needs of Tibetan refugees, to a narrow escape from signing up with the Church Missionary Society to go to Africa (I was barely a theist, let alone a Christian, at the time!). Eventually I found myself being interviewed by Christian Aid for a voluntary post looking after handicapped children in a home run by the Lutheran Church in Austria.

I learnt many things in those five months in Austria, but for present purposes the most important lesson was that there is nothing to fear in mental handicap. Some of the residents in that home looked a little unprepossessing, but I discovered that to be a superficial thing which soon passes as you get to know the individual beneath the unlovely exterior. And many of them had delightful exteriors and some untapped talent as well.

I shall always remember Schnecki, who was remarkably musical. He could pick up any tune with no apparent effort and his party piece, performed in response to 'Schnecki, play/sing Beethoven', was to sing (or pick out on the piano if there was one to hand) faultlessly the theme from the Pastoral Symphony. (Schnecki, by the way, was not Down's, so he does not supply material for the stereotype which classifies all Down's children as musical!)

Not only did I learn not to fear the mentally handicapped, I discovered that they can bring a lot of fun into life, often by puncturing the excessive seriousness of the 'normal' world. An example from Schnecki again. A lady in the village by the name of Frau Braun had recently died and Schnecki had taken this to heart. So, although his vocabulary was limited he knew the word 'died' and the words 'Frau Braun' and tended to associate them very closely. Consequently, in church one Sunday morning, his response to the words in the Creed 'crucified, died...' was a very loud, heartfelt cry of 'Frau Braun!', much to the consternation of the other worshippers. Thereafter, there was some discussion every Sunday morning as to whether it was 'safe' to take Schnecki to church.

Because of my Austrian experience, when Lizzie arrived and it was first tentatively suggested and then confirmed that she had Down's Syndrome, I was spared the fear and the panic that besets many parents of handicapped children, who suddenly feel that they have begotten a monster, a Frankenstein-like cuckoo in the nest, which will stay for ever to shame and frighten them unless they can get shot of it immediately.

There was no anger, no fear, no panic—just an overwhelming sense of sadness. I remember sitting in the small dark room which served as our dining-room, alone in the house because Caroline was still in the hospital, spared by the kindness of my vicar from the usual evening meeting, and brooding. I felt a weight of sadness envelope me, as if I had touched—and in a very small way been touched by—the sadness of the world, perhaps even of God himself. It was not a despairing sadness, in fact there was a sense of purpose and hope within it, a subdued but strong assurance that good would come in time.

When Caroline and Lizzie came home, the routine of life took over once more. For both of us, there was work to be done. For me that meant resuming the life of a curate only recently ordained and only half way through the first year in a large and busy urban parish, a round of preparation, visiting, meetings and more meetings.

Ordination and that first year were traumatic in themselves. I found myself, naturally a rather private person, suddenly a very public person, and very busy too, sometimes from 8 a.m. to 11 p.m., so that my ego was not only exposed but stretched. It was a necessary induction into the realities of ministry. But I longed for privacy and for leisure: just to be able to sit down and do nothing, or sit down and read the paper. The rare occasions when I did get a chance to do these things seemed very precious.

Into this situation came the demands of a new baby, who was moreover handicapped. Very soon we were into the business of working hard at 'stimulating' Lizzie, first with the help of leaflets from the Down's Syndrome Association, and later with Portage charts. It was definitely 'work'.

That, for me, was part of the problem: I had had enough of 'work' and resented it reappearing in this guise. Partly, also, it was ordinary laziness: I felt I had done my bit if I changed a nappy or spooned a bowl of sloppy food into Lizzie's mouth. For the rest I was more interested in making her giggle or attempting to capture her moods with my new camera, the former more successfully than the latter.

Also, I had a suspicion, which I may never have voiced, that underneath all this hard work of stimulating Lizzie there lay a covert attempt to put her 'right', to make up for her handicap by sheer grind, and against that I rebelled, though mostly in the unhelpful fashion of just being bad-tempered and unco-operative about the whole business of Portage. It was worst on holiday: I longed for a day without obligations, schedules and charts to fill in. And it was bad when Lizzie was feeling unco-operative or simply found a particular task very hard. I lacked the patience to coax and teach her and longed just to run with the direction of her inclinations rather than so often against it.

Portage is safely in the past now, much to my relief, and the evidence of her present achievements suggests, without proving beyond doubt, that the early stimulation has had a lot to do with the success she has had. But a doubt persists in my mind. Is the aggression which surfaces sometimes a reaction to having been pushed? Or is it part of her personality? Or is it a side-effect of being almost exclusively in the company of children who are nearly all more able than she is? Or a mixture of all three?

One thing is certain: knowing Lizzie, living under the same roof as Lizzie, being responsible for her as a father—these things have challenged me to the depth of my being. It is sometimes said that after the initial trauma of coming to terms with the fact of your child's handicap, that is the end of the problem. I have found the reverse to be true. Coming to terms with the handicap was the least of my problems. It is living with Lizzie that stretches me.

My upbringing taught me to 'behave' and I have tended to foist that on my children. Lizzie does not always behave. She is quite likely to throw a tantrum, wet her pants (or worse), thump the table or point at a guest and shout, 'She said (or did, or whatever)...' At such moments I forget that Lizzie is handicapped, that people make allowances—and, anyway, so what if they don't!

I would love to be able to say that Lizzie has taught me that outward correctness and a show of good behaviour are not the first priority in life. The truth is that I am just beginning to learn that lesson, which perhaps only Lizzie could have taught me.

It is of course a lesson that might come to any parent from any child, handicapped or not. Often, indeed for most of the time, I forget that Lizzie is handicapped. She is simply part of the family, more infuriating than some, but with her own unique place. And to watch her kicking her football around the yard, fully absorbed and really rather skilful, or gazing fascinated as a mother breastfeeds her baby, or grinning her huge and guileless grin as she decides to forgive you for some way in which you have displeased her—these things are more than enough reward for the struggles along the way.

Two's company?

It was spring—a clear day with blue sky and air smelling fresh with the promise of new life, buds, plants, flowers. I was leaning out of an upstairs window, cleaning off a year's dirt and dust. I idly watched Susie and Nick. They were sitting on logs at the bottom of the garden, logs sawn-up the year before and left to dry out. The daffodils were still bringing their golden light to the middle of the grass, fresh-green and needing to be cut. Nick and Susie were deep in conversation, dressed up partially in cowboy gear. Susie announced that she wanted a gun like Nick's.

I heard Lizzie's voice drifting up from the sitting-room. She wasn't joining her brother and sister outside in the sunshine. She was pronouncing harsh words to her imaginary class again. I knew subconsciously that there would be peace for maybe half-an-hour. I also noted the closeness of Nick and Susie. They rarely argued. If Nick was ill and away from school, there would be peaceful activity from the moment Susie came back from nursery. I didn't like to admit that Lizzie often interfered with their games, but I knew it was true. And yet later that spring morning there were three voices joining in a game of mothers, fathers and babies. There was plenty of amicable discussion.

Relationships are complex and there is no simple description of life between three siblings. Yet I know that Lizzie often plays an argumentative role in their games. Her set ideas and strong personality will clash with the strong ideas of the others. She is less amenable to discussion.

I guess life would be more peaceful if Nick and Susie were left alone to play. But life isn't just about peacefulness. Nick always says that one of his favourite games is playing 'schools' with Lizzie. He also says that when he goes to a new place he feels safe if Lizzie is there too, as she will stick up for him.

Perhaps the clash of temperaments is not simply between Lizzie and the other two. Any two of the children will play more happily together than all three. Sometimes the girls gang up against Nick. Lizzie's aggressiveness is perhaps the hardest thing for the other two to put up with—unless she is defending them against outsiders.

It is impossible to know how different Susie and Nick would have been without Lizzie. I hope that they are more understanding of other children's difficulties and kinder because of it. Lizzie is very possessive about her belongings and is reluctant to share. Susie and Nick are generous. But the fact that Lizzie has often tried to purloin their things does not seem to have had an adverse effect.

I sometimes feel that Nick missed out a bit on my time when he was at the nursery school stage. At that time Lizzie should have been at school full time, but she started nine months later than most children. Nick missed having my undivided attention for part of each day. Yet he has not been pushed out of anything I've done with Lizzie. He has joined in. And now we share a love of books and writing that bonds us together. Mark spends time with Nick, playing chess or wood-working, which they both enjoy.

In any family it is a juggling act to give special time to each child, but we try to do plenty of things together so that no one is left out. In the past we've had to limit activities Lizzie couldn't cope with, but each of them has their own interests now. Nick has music and swimming, Lizzie enjoys the church youth club. Looking back, I think that if anything suffered from lack of time it was my housework, and that doesn't seem such a catastrophe!

Husband and wife

Sometimes there is tension between Mark and me over Lizzie. It is often to do with discipline. I find I put up with more 'bad behaviour' from Lizzie than Mark does—perhaps because of our different personalities. It is especially difficult if Mark is tired and can't tease Lizzie out of her seemingly rude and aggressive responses.

In the past, Portage caused us some pain! But I do not see Lizzie's arrival and presence as ever having a negative influence on our marriage. In the early days, she was a source of sadness, drawing us together as we talked and cried. In later years we have rejoiced together over her achievements, and prayed together about the struggles. I think Lizzie has had a positive effect on our relationship. Perhaps where a marriage suffers from lack of communication, the stress can certainly be great. But difficult times prevent you from papering over the cracks. If there are already problems in a marriage, the arrival of a handicapped child may well be the straw that breaks the camel's back—just like redundancy, illness or any other major stress. Like any other couple, Mark and I have had to sort out our differences, but Lizzie is in no way to blame for the conflicts.

13
Lizzie and Herself

'Mummy, why have I got Down's Syndrome?'

We were driving home from a weekend away. Lizzie woke up, bright as a button after a short sleep. It was dark now and the street lights shone on her glasses as she turned to me and said, 'Mummy, I am mentally handicapped. That is not the same as physically handicapped, is it? That friend, Edward, he is the same as me, and Penny (referring to another friend). Physically handicapped, that means you can't walk...' I smiled at the way Lizzie's thoughts had crystallized over the last few months.

A year ago Lizzie asked lots of questions about what being physically handicapped meant. She had come across several children in wheelchairs when we were on holiday, and she had not been satisfied until I could give a reason for their appearance or problem. She gradually began to understand that she was not physically handicapped, because she could run and walk and 'do things'; but that Down's Syndrome was a mental handicap.

I don't know when Lizzie first heard the name Down's Syndrome but we have always talked openly and if Nick has asked questions we have tried to explain in a way he could understand.

I wanted Lizzie to grow up being totally used to the fact that she has a disability, but also knowing that she is able to overcome it. Yet I wondered if labelling was a good thing. It might make her worried that she couldn't do things when she could.

There were problems for a few months when Lizzie was seven, in the top Infants at school. When she was reprimanded for bad behaviour, she would say, 'I can't help it, I'm handicapped!' She never got away with it, of course.

Lizzie doesn't say that now, but I think there have been times when she has been worried about it. She was frightened when she saw a baby with Down's Syndrome recently. I'm not sure why, but I assume it was because she didn't think that she had once looked like that.

She used to assume that all Down's children wore glasses because she did, and she couldn't understand why people wore glasses when they hadn't got Down's Syndrome. Gradually her classification system has developed enough to include these differences.

Lizzie usually talks about her friends with Down's Syndrome with considerable pride, and she's excluded Nick from some games because he doesn't have Down's Syndrome.

We have tried to talk about it as just one of many problems children can have—not as something that divides people up. I don't know if we have succeeded. The very fact that I am writing this book is an indication that the labelling of people has caused barriers and prejudice that need to be destroyed. For all of us have a tendency to label and classify in a way that separates and divides us. Lizzie is only one member of our family, yet in the book she is highlighted and put under a microscope.

I've said that Lizzie's tendency to think all Down's children wear glasses is because her classification system is not very well developed. Yet there are plenty of adults— without that excuse—who make gross generalizations about Down's children. These generalizations are passed on to the general public and then back to parents of babies with Down's Syndrome who then, like us, have to spend the next few years unlearning and exploding the myths and labels with all that they imply. It annoyed me to hear on the television recently that common stereotype of a young Down's child:

'She's so loving.' I suddenly felt angry. Lizzie isn't always loving to her friends or to her brother and sister. If she is tired she can be spiteful—like any other child. Do we have to believe Down's children are loving in order to value them? Can't we value them, like everyone else, just for being here?

So how does Lizzie see herself? In the past she has suffered from a sense of inferiority, a feeling that too much is expected of her. The Portage project, while giving me support in the early years and a structured way of helping her—so helpful at first—may also have contributed to a tendency towards unreal expectations and goal-setting based entirely on behaviour. We lose the varied patterns of development and interest in children if we try to fit them into a system. Are we loving them for themselves when we are looking to see if they have learnt a particular skill? In highlighting what they can't do, and what needs to be taught, we can lose sight of them simply as children—good at some things and not good at others.

I do not measure Nick and Susie's progress every six months. I do try to encourage them in the things that interested them. I never get very worried about things they don't like. But Lizzie was made to learn things she was not interested in because the skill appeared on the checklist. I felt she might not learn it otherwise. Every skill was taught in the prescribed order to begin with, until we learnt to be more flexible.

Because of my own sense of inadequacy about whether I could teach Lizzie successfully, and where I was in coming to grips with her handicap, I was unable simply to use Portage as the tool it is meant to be. I was too emotionally involved. It is a very helpful tool, as long as we see it simply as a tool and do not become enslaved to it. Parents need confidence in their child to use the Portage project effectively. This develops in time, but anxiety can get in the way.

Early intervention programmes are known to help Down's children in many ways but there is current debate, in academic circles at least, about what is most effective in

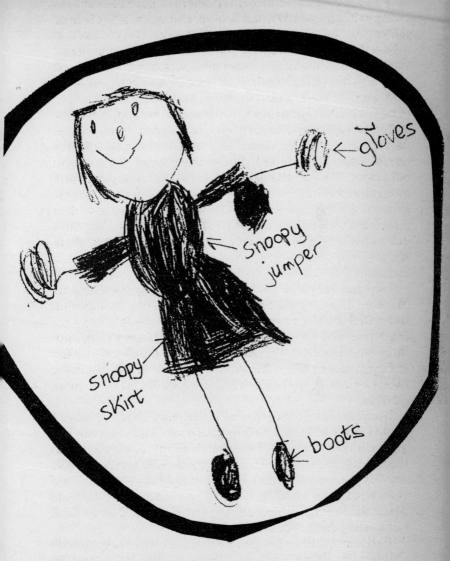

A drawing of Lizzie by herself: aged 8³/4.

nurturing handicapped children and helping them fulfil their potential. Which is more important—a loving, accepting parent without a structured programme, or a programme alone? Is a structured programme really necessary? Or is informed, affirming parenting just as effective? The best of both worlds would seem to be to use a programme, but have the kind of flexible approach that puts it in perspective. But first-time around parents like ourselves need very skilled counselling to make this possible.

Parents need to be aware of children's needs at each age and to feel able to meet those needs—intellectually and socially. But children don't learn if they are unhappy and they don't learn if too much pressure is put on them, or if they sense that they are loved only if they are successful.

As I have learnt to love and accept Lizzie more, my sights have been lowered in some areas—and then she has often surprised me.

On the other hand, I have often expected her to enjoy something and she has found it too hard. After some fruitless efforts to get her to a gym class, I realized that she couldn't cope and didn't enjoy it, so it was better left alone.

Lizzie likes to know where she is and finds new situations quite difficult. This is reflected in her enjoyment of tidying her room and in wanting to talk through each day the night before, asking what we will do at every stage.

In the family, Lizzie is very competitive, perhaps because she is aware that the others can do things she can't or perhaps out of natural sibling rivalry.

All children have a strong sense of justice, especially if they feel they've been done out of anything. Lizzie quickly gets upset if Nick goes to play with one of his friends and she hasn't someone to play with herself.

We have wondered about Lizzie's bossy, controlling behaviour. Did she boss Edward because she was surrounded by children more able than herself at school, and had no chance to be the organizer? But she organizes activities at home sometimes. So her bossiness may be her nature, because she has a strong personality, not because she is compensating for something.

There is no doubt that as Lizzie has moved into a happier, more settled and mature phase, she has gained a good self-image. In the conversation I recorded, I discovered she felt she was kind and helpful, tall, slim, pretty and good at all her work. Not bad!

Lizzie is beginning to enjoy wearing more grown-up clothes and often puts on my make-up and perfume. She likes to choose her own clothes to wear and takes pride in her appearance.

But her self-worth grows most through being loved, and our talk, cuddle and prayer last thing at night when she is tucked up in bed and about to go to sleep—is important to both of us. She often begins, 'Mummy I want to tell you something.' Sometimes she will tell me things she has been worried about, like being upset about being bullied at school. Lizzie and I sometimes talk about what she would like to do when she is grown up. Sometimes she wants to be a nursery-nurse and look after babies; she loves babies.

School has helped her self-image to develop. She is treated like the other children and expected to behave properly. No one talks about her being different. To learn to love others is to learn to respect them. The only way Lizzie can have a good self-image is in feeling this respect from the people around her. Lizzie does feel loved. There may have been times in the past when she hasn't.

When Lizzie really wanted an answer to her question 'Mummy, why have I got Down's Syndrome?', I always used to reply 'Because God made you that way.' I assume Lizzie was satisfied with that answer because she doesn't ask the question at the moment. I hope too that she thinks it is fine to have Down's Syndrome, so it doesn't matter if she has it or not.

Recently, Lizzie had to go into hospital for a minor exploratory operation. She claimed the bed she wanted to sleep in and then went off to play on an old-fashioned wooden rocking horse in the playroom (the sort we always wanted as children). The operation was due the next day. In a side-room I discovered there was a new-born baby who had Down's Syndrome. As soon as Lizzie heard about the baby, she wanted to hold and feed him. The nurse and I talked: the baby was to be fostered because his parents didn't feel they could take him home. Lizzie sat on a chair and the tiny baby nestled into her arms. He had downy dark hair and delicate features. I said, almost unconsciously, 'What a shame.' Lizzie immediately said, 'What's the matter with him?'

'Well,' I said uneasily, 'He's got Down's Syndrome...and he can't feed very well.'

'But what is the matter with him?' she asked again. And I could see that, in in her eyes, Down's Syndrome did not count as something wrong.

I was glad Lizzie saw things that way. Yet I knew my answer to her question, 'God made you that way', was unsatisfactory. Down's Syndrome *was* 'something wrong'. The answer might satisfy Lizzie, but it wasn't enough. Why did God allow children to be born imperfect, with brains that did not function properly and bodies that didn't work efficiently? Lizzie was healthy and able in many ways, but what about the children who were much more severely handicapped? Why?

There is no easy answer. The problem as I see it goes right back to the roots of human history.

The message of the early chapters of the Bible's book of Genesis is clear: when men and women turn away from God and choose to go their own way, things go wrong. In the terms of the story, they have to leave the Garden, a place of safety and security. The man's job becomes difficult, hard labour. The woman's experience of child-birth is painful. Pain and suffering enter human experience. Perfection is spoiled.

Everything that is wrong in the world—the evils of suffering and sickness, and the hurt we inflict on one another—comes from a world at odds with itself and its

Creator. People are alienated from the very Being with whom they should feel most 'at home'.

Suffering, sickness, things going wrong, are the common human experience. Bad things happen to all of us, simply because we are part of a world that is marred.

But God is good. He doesn't want suffering or sickness in the world. He loves us, his creation. He hurts with our hurt. He cries with our tears. God doesn't want a world marred, but he made people, not robots. God gave us free will and, in giving us choice, God risked rebellion. We have to *choose* to follow him. Wrong choices bring their own consequences. But God did not leave the world to stew in its own juice. He came himself, in the person of his Son, Jesus Christ, to sort out the mess. By his life and death and resurrection he paid for our rebellion and opened the way to forgiveness and a new life—ultimately to a new creation altogether. In the short-term, pain and suffering are not wiped out, but they can be transformed.

I don't believe God wanted Lizzie or anyone else to be handicapped. But because we live in an imperfect world, handicap happens. God *allows* it to happen. The only way we can make sense of it is to accept it, not as the result of the machinations of some Being who wants to punish us, but as the gift of a loving Father. In accepting Lizzie as God's gift to us we can let God transform the situation into something better than it would have been otherwise. So in that sense, yes, God did make Lizzie the way she is.

This is no glib answer to the problem of suffering. This way of thinking does not come easily, but it yields its own fruit of personal growth, peace and even gratitude that God has given us so much.

14
Being Lizzie's Mum

For the first five years or so of Lizzie's life I was very aware of every bit of her progress or lack of it. I tested her out. I had wanted to know what she knew.

My own learning has been partly a process of self-acceptance and partly one of getting to know Lizzie in a way that meant I could love and accept her—as she is.

Acceptance of ourselves takes a long time to develop and it can be held back by false expectations.

How Not To Be A Perfect Mum is the title of a book written recently by radio presenter and author Libby Purves. The need for a book like this is obvious. We all come to motherhood with an image we aspire to. It can be based on all kinds of models. I aspired to the model of an ever-calm, kind, peaceful parent, and the anger I felt towards Lizzie when she was unpredictable or badly behaved was hard to reconcile with that. I had to learn my own limitations and be able to accept my failures.

One nightmare experience returns to me every time I get off the escalator at the top of Birmingham New Street station and walk into the shopping area.

One Easter I decided to take Lizzie and Nick by train to Wolverhampton to see my sister. Nick was nearly two and Lizzie was four at the time. We had to change at New Street station. I decided to take them to the Early Learning Centre to play, while we waited for the next train. While we were there Nick needed to use the toilet. I asked in the Centre, but we were not allowed to use the staff loo and I was directed to the public toilets in the shopping area. I didn't want to take Lizzie with me because she was likely to play around or run off; it seemed more sensible to leave her to read her beloved Postman Pat books in the Centre. I thought she would be safe there. How foolish I was.

When I returned with Nick, Lizzie had vanished. I felt sick with fear. What could have happened to her? I asked the assistants and their answers did not help. 'She went out with another family.' That made the situation worse. I rushed out to find a security man. He was kind and said he would alert the shops.

I looked everywhere, clutching Nick, a heavy toddler, in my arms. Eventually the security man came up to me again, after I'd been in and out of several shops. 'I think you'd better prepare yourself,' he said. I felt desperate by now. What on earth had happened?

I walked into an electrical store. There, in front of a row of amazed assistants, was Lizzie, with no clothes on and a large pooh on the floor.

Behind me came a line of rubber-gloved women, armed with black plastic bags. I was scarlet with embarrassment, upset, but very relieved. The security man told me not to worry, they would clear it up. I dressed Lizzie rapidly and rushed out of the shop, shaking. We made our way to the waiting train and I dropped into a seat. I didn't know whether to laugh or cry, but in the end laughter won. Yet even now I can't go near that Early Learning Centre without feeling sick.

I had failed to look after my child properly. It does happen. We are all liable to misjudge and make mistakes. We are subject to pressures. Human beings are not perfect. Why should any mother be an expert at child rearing—something for which none of us is trained before we are launched into it. I've had to forgive myself so often for getting angry and being unkind; I've had to ask the children to forgive me too. I've had to hang on to the fact that God forgives me.

The Christian gospel is about our acceptance by God, because he loves us with no strings attached. Unconditional love is a love we find hard to give and to receive, for many reasons, but it does become possible as we learn to be more patient with ourselves and to have mercy on our failures. Perhaps it's our pride that makes so many of us expect to be perfect.

Another important element in accepting ourselves is being able to acknowledge our real feelings about something.

I met a mother who had adopted a Down's child at eighteen months. She was eager to talk to me. Her child was now ten and she was struggling to get a place for her in mainstream school. Yet her real problem was the difficulty she had in forgiving the anger she felt towards her child. She admitted to me the hateful, negative feelings we find it so hard to speak about. We know the answer is not to smack, but to hold our child tightly; but sometimes the feeling of anger wins, and then the sense of guilt at being a bad mother overwhelms us. There are things we don't really wish to happen but the thoughts are there in our head. There are the words we yell, hoping against hope that no one hears us. In this situation, what we can do is pray, as that woman and I prayed—offering her child to God. We can hear God saying 'I will carry this burden for you' and find comfort and strength in his promise.

One of my friends who has an autistic child used to go and scream in her bedroom when everything got too much—to let out the anger and frustration. We so often refuse to acknowledge our anger because we want to protect the image we have of ourselves. Yet in acknowledging the dark side of ourselves, in realising that it exists in all of us, we can receive peace and healing.

God loves us and wants us to let him into our lives. It is no good waiting until we feel good enough before we come to him. We have to come now. We will never be good enough but he loves us as we are, he will always love us, and he offers us forgiveness and help.

Why do we find it so hard to believe that God really does accept us, warts and all? Even those who are Christians, who

138

have committed themselves to God, still often behave as if God will only love them if they are good.

As I have grasped the truth of God's love for me more fully, I have been able to love Lizzie more too. And my love for her has grown as I have learnt who she is.

You may know the story of Dibs, the child who did not speak and who behaved as if he was mentally retarded—yet was perfectly normal. The book, *Dibs in Search of Self*, records these shocking and moving words:

'The psychiatrist told us...that Dibs was not mentally defective or psychotic or brain-damaged, but the most rejected and emotionally deprived child he had ever seen. He said that my husband and I were the ones who needed the help...'

Dibs underwent psychotherapy for about a year, when he was five. There he was able to express how he really felt and he was able to grow towards normality. He received affirmation and respect in this experience and his parents began to understand him.

His mother tried to put her own feelings into words: 'I had to prove something to myself...I had to prove that he could learn, I had to prove that I could teach him. And yet his behaviour was such that I never knew how much got through to him or how much it all meant. I would watch him bend over the things I had given him when he was alone in his room and I would say to myself, "He wouldn't do this if it meant nothing to him." And yet I was never sure.'

I was moved by a sense of familiarity as I read the book. Dibs was not Lizzie, and I was not his mother...and yet...

To love someone is to respect them. If we don't understand someone we can't respect them. When Lizzie couldn't speak or explain what she felt or why she did things, it was hard to know what she was thinking. (It was like a stroke patient who has so much to express yet is unable to articulate the words.) Yet when I imposed on her a learning programme and activities I felt were 'good' for her I was not respecting her wants and desires. It was partly that I didn't know what they were, but often I thought that what Lizzie wanted to do would not 'teach' her anything. I sometimes needed to wait for Lizzie's time. Lizzie needs space, space to play on her own, space not to be controlled. In this she is like her sister and her father.

I watch Lizzie today, out of the kitchen window, as I wash up. She kicks her football around the small patio enclosed by walls and then rides her new pink bike. She is happy. Some times she talks to herself, sometimes she sings. Or later she may go upstairs to her room and organize 'schools'. 'Now, are you all settled?' she says to her imaginary children. She needs space. She can be trusted now to use it sensibly.

On walks in a nearby Country Park, Lizzie will often wander off a little way from where we are sitting or playing and come back later, happier. Now she is older she can be trusted to come back. She might not have done so a few years ago.

As Lizzie has grown older and become able to organize games she enjoys, it has been easier to let her develop on her own. I have sometimes felt frustrated as I cleared up after a complicated game of 'going to college', and yet I can't help enjoying her plastic bag carefully packed with a toothbrush, sponge, soap and clothes; her table next to the settee laid with a clock and her Bible, notebook and pen.

At Christmas and birthdays I am always struck by Lizzie's lack of acquisitiveness. All she ever asks for is a grown-up box of chocolates with what they contain on the lid, and a packet of felt pens. She always receives these, and other things besides. I find it touching that she is satisfied with such simple things. I was pleased she actually wanted a bicycle for her birthday this year.

She enjoys things for what they are, and she either likes a thing or she doesn't. So many of the educational toys I used to buy her were untouched—until Nick or Susie came along—because she didn't enjoy them. Things she enjoys are played with endlessly like her organ, her dolls, her pens and writing-books.

140

If I really respect her I must let her choose. The conflict, often, is how to help Lizzie choose sensibly without her feeling that the choice is made for her. As our confidence in her understanding grows, it is easier to leave the choices to her. As our relationship has blossomed I have noticed that Lizzie is more sensitive to my being cross with her. She is very upset if she thinks I'm cross with her, and it is far easier now to reason with her. Stickers to reward good behaviour really do act as an incentive and help her choose to co-operate.

She still likes me to sit on the landing and read while she goes to sleep, and these days I usually comply. I feel I have often rejected her needs in the past and been too forceful. I want to build up her security now. Because I feel much happier about my relationship with Lizzie I feel more relaxed, and this in turn feeds into the relationship. An upward spiral is created, rather than a downward one.

It is hard to separate my acceptance of Lizzie from her own growing out of the egocentric phase which I found so difficult. Yet decisions I made in the past to hold and cuddle her, and now to offer her to God nightly for him to heal and help and fill with his Spirit, also play an important part.

I first heard about the 'holding technique' in connection with therapy for autistic children, yet I could see the links with Lizzie's behaviour. Just after our last move, there was a time when Lizzie wouldn't look at me when I held her, and she didn't seem to want me to kiss her or say I loved her or that she was lovely. However, I persevered, and gradually over a period of weeks she began to respond. I would hold her gently but firmly at bathtime every night for a few minutes and tell her to look at me. Gradually she did, and I felt a change in her responses. Her bolshiness became less and our relationship improved.

In the end it seems that all these factors merge together. I believe that God uses all things to work together for good. Lizzie now feels good about herself. She is pleased with the fact that she can read and write. She can express her needs and feelings, and she can be independent to some extent.

I know too that I can only do my best. I will never be a perfect Mum—and I don't have to be. So there is a mutual acceptance and respect.

Acceptance of people and situations does not mean we abdicate responsibility, or stop seeking to help in the best possible way, but what does change is our level of anxiety about the outcome. I may decide to ignore extreme rudeness because Lizzie is very tired. I may decide to cuddle her instead. Mercy is perhaps more important than principle.

After we have tried to do our best, we can leave the outcome with God. We no longer have anything to prove.

I recently read a meditation in Jean Vanier's book, *The Broken Body*. It seemed to mirror my experience:

'You are called to accept and integrate your darkness and your brokenness, letting the healing Spirit of Jesus penetrate into those parts of your being where you are so terribly vulnerable and even frightened. He knows us so well, for he is the Word who created us. He alone can make all things new, out of wisdom and love, as the Creator. It is only as you become whole, as you accept your own brokenness and misery and as you let the healing power and mercy of Jesus, our Saviour, descend upon you, and rise within you, that you will become a source of unity for others. It is only if you discover your thirst and drink of Jesus, that you can flow over into others, giving peace.

'So let us open ourselves to the healing, forgiving Spirit of Jesus...'

15
Lizzie 'Taking Flight'

When Lizzie was in hospital and met the Down's baby, the issue of parents rejecting their handicapped children was raised again. I couldn't tell Lizzie the real reason why that baby was on the ward. But I would have loved his parents to have met Lizzie. The nurses said that too: Lizzie was a real hit with them. And they were sweet to her, making her extra toast, letting her help them at the desk when she couldn't go to sleep and I had to go home. I think she entertained them by her very direct questions and comments. She made frequent visits to the baby's room and would pick him up and wind him, holding him over her shoulder as if she'd done it for years. A confident girl and a fragile tiny baby—drawn together by a kind of magnetism. Just after Lizzie was born I would have felt angry with the baby's parents. Now I understood better the pain they experienced. But I felt very sad—sad for *them*, because I felt their lives would be the poorer if they tried to live as if this momentous event had never happened. How could they really come to terms with something they were trying to forget? Forgetting is not healing.

A journalist for *The Independent* wrote an article entitled 'When baby isn't perfect'. She spoke of the expectation that in the latter part of the twentieth century we can all produce perfect babies, and went on to say: 'Medical advances have left parents ill-equipped to cope, particularly when babies are born months premature. As the numbers of children born with defects falls in the coming decades, parents and society at large may find it increasingly difficult to accept handicap. This will make it even more important for us to recognize the desperation of a diminishing number of families with an ''imperfect'' child. We must learn to understand their confusion and also to welcome the idea that children who are different enrich our lives.'

One thing I think could help in my own area is something that is already done elsewhere to great effect. Parent-groups are trained in counselling skills and make themselves available to visit new parents of handicapped children. A member of such a group can come alongside the new parents, not in a judgmental manner, but to share the pain being suffered and to answer any questions that might help them have the confidence to begin their life with their child.

One Sunday evening recently, the telephone rang. I got up from the settee rather reluctantly to answer it. Mark was at church. Susannah was asleep. The older children had just had a bath and we were in the sitting-room, reading stories before bedtime. I prized these times and disliked the intrusion. Yet as the unfamiliar voice at the other end of the phone began to talk, I was interested. Were we busy? Could they come over now, and bring the baby? Could they see Lizzie? 'Of course you can,' I replied and put the phone down.

I was strangely excited. The children picked up my feelings and decided they would both have to wait up for the visitors. A few more stories later, the doorbell rang and the family arrived.

My visitors were the couple I had gone to see in the special baby-care unit of the hospital a few months before. No longer pale faced, a smiling woman entered the sitting room and her husband followed, carrying a Moses basket. I peered in. The little girl was no longer red in the reflected hospital lights but a healthy colour. I picked her up, still light and tiny, but responsive too.

Lizzie had hidden behind the rocking-chair, overcome by

144

shyness. She seemed worried. She wouldn't come out and see the baby. I couldn't decide what she was worried about. She knew the baby had Down's Syndrome. Maybe she found it hard to think there had been a time when she was as tiny and helpless as this little girl.

Embarrassment slowly evaporated as I tried to explain that Lizzie was tired and a bit shy. Soon she was out of her hiding-place and joining Nick, who was shaking toys for the baby to watch.

The parents told me they had left their daughter in the hospital for a few painful weeks, but had soon felt compelled to bring her home. They hadn't regretted their decision. The rejection they had made out of fear, grief and shock had turned to acceptance. But they would not have an easy ride. Their daughter needed heart surgery and would take a long time to put on weight. Even so, they had decided that they couldn't opt out. They couldn't leave her to someone else.

The struggle that all parents of handicapped children have is not primarily with the child, although there are bound to be conflicts. The real struggle is an internal one: the struggle to come to terms with what has happened, or to reject it. Rejecting can take the form of denying the problem—failing to acknowledge the child's limitations—rather than actual rejection of the child.

'Normalization', is a popular theme today. It is spoken of a great deal in the context of educating handicapped children. Helping children to fulfil their own special potential, to be as 'normal', as like their peers, as they can, is good. But we cannot make children un-handicapped. If total 'normality' is our goal, we may be failing to accept the value of our children in themselves. We may be saying they are not acceptable unless they are 'normal'. That is a kind of rejection.

Parents feel anger at their child's limitations. Often we confuse our anger at the handicap with anger at the child. Anger is a powerful force. It is often projected onto people inappropriately, because otherwise we might turn it on ourselves. When I was angry with Lizzie over her failure to get potty trained, I knew deep-down that it wasn't her fault. Yet my feelings had nowhere to go except inward on myself or outwards to her. If I had had access to a non-judgmental counsellor it might have helped. Some health authorities are successfully using the idea of a 'key worker', who is placed with a family from the birth of their child onwards: available to talk through any problems if the parents ask.

Dealing with the anger can help to prevent the development of rejection and resentment against the child. Growing to respect and understand our children often takes time. I can see now that some of my own most difficult conflicts with Lizzie have been times when I've intruded too much into her personal space and freedom. I've been too controlling. Lizzie has fought back to preserve her identity.

Lizzie needs help and guidance to live appropriately, but she also needs freedom to choose and the balance is a fine one. She needs help to understand that stealing is wrong, and that crossing roads is dangerous, unless done carefully. But I can give her freedom to choose her own clothes, and I'd like her to do so.

Lizzie has an ability to remember which we all respect. She reminded Mark and me about Valentine's Day this year. She managed to remind Mark about the card she had helped him choose a few days before, without telling me about it beforehand or letting me know on the day.

Forthcoming events like the School Disco are never forgotten, and her independence at the most recent one put me firmly in my place. I was concerned that Lizzie would lose her refreshment money as she had no pocket. 'It's OK Mum,' she said very firmly as I hovered around before the Disco started, suggesting she could give the money to her teacher. She obviously wanted me to leave. When I picked her up later she told me she had given the change to another teacher to look after and proudly gave it me back. She could cope.

It is easy to respect her independence and also to enjoy the love and acceptance she gives us. Lizzie is best appreciated when we are one to one (something that is true of many

146

children). I had to fetch her from school recently, leaving the other two ill at home. Lizzie's enjoyment of a walk to the shops to collect something on the way home, and her happy chatter, was therapeutic.

She is faithful and loving, accepting us totally. When I feel frayed at the edges, a hug from Lizzie makes me feel loved. All our children do this. But there seems a paradoxical selflessness about Lizzie, especially when she knows she has one of us on her own.

Lizzie does not bear grudges and is very forgiving, but she is very naughty sometimes and she knows how to wind people up and annoy them. She can be merciless in doing this to Nick or Susie, and gives a good thump or kick if need be.

So I wonder what people mean when they talk about the eternal innocence of Down's children. Perhaps it is the fact that they seem to be without malicious intent. They do not wish evil on anyone. Yet I sometimes I feel that talking of 'eternal innocence' is like saying 'they are so loving'— providing a reason for loving and accepting Down's children, rather than loving and accepting them for who they are: people made in God's image, like the rest of us.

Jean Vanier has much to say about acceptance and rejection. He believes that the mentally disabled have many gifts to share with those around them and that they are not the people most afflicted in society:

'The greatest suffering is not an afflicted person... What is serious is a heart that was made to love and does not. The suffering of our men does not come from encephalitis or meningitis or the fact that their mother had German measles... It is the fact that they are rejected, that is the worst thing. The greatest affliction is to reject someone. It is even greater than to be rejected. It is a terrible sickness of the heart.'

As I have read more about Jean Vanier's L'Arche communities I have begun to understand more fully what

147

accepting and respecting another human being, simply because they are human, is about.

The handicapped people in these communities have no possessions or status. They are the epitome of the 'poor' as described in the Old and New Testaments. The Bible says over and over again that God has a special place for the poor and disadvantaged:

'God stands at the right hand of the needy one, to save his life from those who condemn him' (Psalm 109).

'I know that the Lord secures justice for the poor, and upholds the cause of the needy' (Psalm 140).

'He who despises his neighbour sins, but blessed is he who is kind to the needy' (Proverbs 14:21).

'He who oppresses the poor shows contempt for their Maker, but whoever is kind to the needy honours God' (Proverbs 14:31).

Jean Vanier speaks of hardness of the heart being the greatest sin. Proverbs 21 says, 'If a man shuts his ears to the cry of the poor he too will cry out and not be answered.'

The New Testament also speaks of the weak and poor:

'Blessed are the poor in spirit for theirs is the kingdom of heaven. Blessed are the meek, for they shall inherit the earth. Blessed are you when people insult you, persecute you and falsely say all kinds of evil against you because of me. Rejoice and be glad, because great is your reward in heaven...' (Matthew 5).

'When you have a banquet, invite the poor, the crippled, the lame, the blind, and you will be blessed. Although they cannot repay you, you will be repaid at the resurrection of the righteous' (Luke 14).

And James in his letter writes: 'has not God chosen those who are poor in the eyes of the world to be rich in faith and to inherit the kingdom he promised to those who love him? But you have insulted the poor...'

There are biblical principles here. If we honour the 'poor', we will be honoured, because whatever we do to others we are doing to Christ.

Yet so much of our treatment of handicapped and disadvantaged people does not honour them. It segregates and hides them, and it deprives them of parental love and affection. It denies them the right to an appropriate education and proper significance in life. We may have done this out of ignorance or fear, but we have also done it because these people cannot answer back. We have encouraged the aborting of imperfect children. We have made it easy for parents to reject their newborn babies. We have supported the idea of bussing children several miles from home to segregated schools. We have encouraged others to hide these problems away. We have encouraged it if we have not spoken out against it, if we have been uncaring by not getting involved.

Loving and respecting or honouring people has to be learned. Our values sometimes have to be questioned and changed—and this is difficult. Lizzie has commanded our respect by her tenacity and courage to battle on, to learn to write, to read, and to swim.

Suffering is part of life, and without it we do not grow up. Although our personal suffering may appear small and insignificant compared with other traumas and loss, to us it has meaning because through it we have been changed.

Coming to terms with labels, a sense of failure, an aloneness at the beginning that we felt few shared, a sense of loss and then our own limited patience, has brought us to the end of our own resources. We have had to realize, too, that having a child who does not look or behave in the way we initially wanted does not show that we are inadequate or failures. We have had to let God rebuild our self-image.

The last three years have been good for us in this respect as well as for Lizzie. We have not had the careful assessments, case conferences and recommendations that were conscientiously produced in our previous home, perhaps. The involvement of professionals can sometimes create dependency and a sense of inadequacy in parents, even if this is not intended.

Lizzie's placement at a school where the head has had confidence in her has helped us all to feel confident. There have been no assessments. Although her progress is monitored generally, the magnifying glass has been removed and we have all learnt to breathe more freely.

So Lizzie is being launched into independence, slowly but surely. She is a little bird with clipped wings but she is beginning to fly strongly. Her flight has been aided by the warmth and love and respect of her teachers at school, her friends, our church family, and also her own determination.

Lizzie wants a job, a boyfriend, a marriage and even a baby when she is older. It is a long time until then but I wonder what right anyone has to deny her these things. She will have worked hard for them like anyone else if they become hers one day.

A book is bound to be an inadequate means to describe a faithful, pretty, lively, mischievous little girl. But this book has not simply been about Lizzie. It has been about a love affair between a mother and a daughter, a father, a brother and a sister—a family. Most love affairs are stormy, there is anger and disappointment, resolution and joy.

When Lizzie hugs me and says 'I love you, Mummy,' that is enough. In receiving her love, I also receive the love of the God who gave her to us.

APPENDIX

1. What is Down's Syndrome?

Down's Syndrome occurs in one out of every 700 live births a year, more commonly to mothers over forty-five, when the risk of a Down's baby is a one in five chance.

Down's Syndrome is called Trisomy 21 because there is an extra chromosome 21. It is thought that the translocation occurs at conception when the cells divide, when the egg is ageing and is more likely to be unstable—hence the higher incidence in older women.

The extra chromosome affects physical features (all are not necessarily present in each child): an epicanthic fold under the eyes, a single crease on the palm of the hand, flattened nose, smaller than normal head, shorter arms and—because of hypotonic muscles—often a tongue that protrudes out of a smaller than average mouth. There are often gut or heart defects. There are mental effects too: language development is impaired and there is general mental retardation of varying degrees. A few children have mosaic Down's Syndrome, where not all the cells have an extra chromosome. About 3 per cent have hereditary Down's Syndrome.

2. The Down's Syndrome Association

The Down's Syndrome Association is the leading organization for helping parents and professionals with the care, treatment and training of children with Down's Syndrome. It has a resource centre in London and a research centre in Birmingham, a dozen branches and scores of self-help groups. It has a sister organization in the Scottish Down's Syndrome Association.

The DSA was founded in 1970 as a result of the efforts of Rex Brinkworth, a child psychologist who demonstrated that Down's children are less handicapped if they are given extra stimulation and training from the very earliest age.

How can the DSA help?

○ By encouraging new parents to embark on a detailed programme of stimulation, exercise and diet to bring out the very best in their child—a potential much greater than used to be thought.

○ By providing a counselling service for the parents at a time of shock and distress.

○ By setting up local self-help groups so that parents can share their problems and help each other to adopt a positive approach to solving them.

○ By providing information and advice about education, teenage problems, life after school, leaving home and housing.

○ By promoting and carrying out research into ways of diminishing the effects of Down's Syndrome.

○ By creating greater public awareness of the potential of Down's children, a more sympathetic understanding of their needs and greater respect for their right to lead fulfilling and useful lives.

The Association believes that the mere presence of Down's Syndrome in a new-born baby is not a sufficient reason for allowing the child to die.

The Down's Syndrome Association has a literature list which covers a wide range of relevant topics.

For further information contact:

The Down's Syndrome Association, Head Office, 153-155 Mitcham Road, Tooting, London SW17 9PG *Tel.* 081 682 4001

The National Centre for Down's Syndrome, Room 154, Birmingham Polytechnic, Westbourne Road, Edgbaston, Birmingham B15 5TN. (The DSA sponsors this research centre.)

3. Advice on education

The following organizations are of help to parents regarding the education of their child and provide help and support in the statement process and advice on integration:

ACE (The Advisory Centre for Education), 18 Victoria Park Square, London EZ9 PB *Tel.* 081 980 4596

The Children's Legal Centre, 20 Compton Terrace, London N1 2UN
Tel. 071 359 6251 (2–5 p.m.)

CSIE (The Centre for Studies on Integration in Education), 415 Edgware
Road, London NW2 6NB   *Tel.* 081 452 8642

IPSEE (The Independent Panel of Special Education Experts),
Administrator: John Wright, 12 Marsh Road, Tillingham, Essex CM0 7SZ
Tel. 0621 87 781. Registered Office: 20 Compton Terrace, London N1 2UN
    This charity provides parents, free of charge, with expert second opinions
on their child's learning difficulties and on the appropriateness or otherwise of
the educational provision on offer.

The Rathbone Society, 1st Floor, Princess House, 105/107 Princess Street,
Manchester
    This organization produces literature helpful when seeking to make a
parental contribution to the statement.

Voluntary Council for Handicapped Children, 8 Wakely Street, London
EC1V 7QE   *Tel.* 071 278 9441
    This organization has a free information and a range of publications such as
a reading list on special educational needs and an invaluable list of
organizations concerned with specific disabilities or difficulties in learning.

4. Parent groups

Network 81, Membership Secretary: Elizabeth Arrondelle, 52, Magnaville
Road, Bishop's Stortford, Herts CM23 4DW   *Tel.* 0279 503244
    This is a growing national network of support groups run by and for parents
whose children have disabilities or learning difficulties.

CASE (Campaign for the Advancement of State Education)—information
from: Sue Hodgson, The Grove, 110 High Street, Sawston, Cambs CB2 4HJ
Tel. 0223 833179

5. Portage

This pre-school education project provides a great deal of practical help for
parents, plus weekly activity charts. Useful books (see Bibliography below)
can be obtained from:

NFER, Nelson Danille House, 2 Oxford Road East, Windsor, Berks SL4 1DF

6. Life after school

Christian Concern for the Mentally Handicapped
A Cause for Concern, PO Box 351, Reading, Berks RG17 AL
Tel. 0734 508781

This organization provides long-term residential homes for handicapped adults, which are church-linked. See also the Directory of Residential Accommodation for the Mentally Handicapped, published by MENCAP, 1982. Available at public libraries and from MENCAP. A Cause for Concern also provides useful study material for church groups and others: a publications list is available from headquarters.

7. Lichfield Diocesan Study Group

Lichfield Diocesan Committee, Diocesan Office, St Mary's House, The Close, Lichfield, Staffs

The study group has produced a useful pack for churches about people with a mental handicap called 'God Made me Too', produced by the Lichfield Diocesan Committee for People with a Mental Handicap.

8. Kaleidoscope Drama and Arts Centre

Kaleidoscope Drama and Arts Centre, 19 Mellish Road, Walsall, West Midlands WS4 2DQ

Kaleidoscope is seeking to establish a national residential drama and arts centre for mentally handicapped young people. It tours England and Europe with productions using both ablebodied and handicapped actors.

9. Professional help

Sue Buckley, Portsmouth Down's Syndrome Trust, Dept of Psychology, Portsmouth Polytechnic, King Charles Street, Portsmouth PO1 2ER

The trust provides weekends for parents with opportunities to discuss problems with professionals.

10. Advice on heart problems

The Down's Heart Group, 48 Main Street, Lyddington, Rutland

This group, founded by Linda Walsh, has been set up to help families whose Down's child has heart problems. There are groups now throughout the country, with regional contacts.

11. Useful resources

The following are some of the books, games and computer programmes that I have found useful in helping Lizzie at home.

BOOKS ENJOYED PRE-SCHOOL:

Alan and Janet Ahlberg, *Each Peach, Pear, Plum* and *Peepo*, Penguin. (The rhyming quality and design of these books encourage involvement.)

Heather Amery and Stephen Cartwright, *The First 1000 Words*, Usborne.

Raymond Briggs, *The Snowman*. Jan Ormerod, *Moonlight* and *Sunshine*, Picture Puffins. (These three books are text-less picture books and encourage the child's involvement in telling the story.)

Eric Carle, *The Very Hungry Caterpillar*, Picture Puffin. (A good number book and useful for days of the week.)

Roger Hargreaves, *The Mr Men Books*, World International Publications. (These are enjoyed for their clear drawings and humour.)

Eric Hill, *Spot's First Walk, Spot's First Christmas, Spot Goes to School, Spot's Birthday*, Picture Puffins. (Flap books encourage participation by the child.)

Shirley Hughes, *Dogger* and *Helpers*, Bodley Head. *Lucy and Tom Go to the Seaside*, Gollancz.

Topsy and Tim stories, Blackie—like Shirley Hughes' books, these are enjoyed for their familiar, family-based topics.

Jill Murphy, *Peace at Last, Five Minutes Peace, Whatever Next!*, Macmillan.

Elfrida Vipont and Raymond Briggs, *The Elephant and the Bad Baby*, Hamish Hamilton.

BOOKS LIZZIE CAN BEGIN TO READ HERSELF:

Bill Gillham, Methuen Paired Reading Storybooks—*Awful Arrabella, Our Baby Bites, Our Baby Throws Things* and others.

Ladybird Read It Yourself series, for example: *The Three Bears* and others.

BOOKS WE READ TOGETHER:

R. Carlisle and L. Wendon, *Letterland*, Hamlyn/Templar. (Excellent for teaching letters of the alphabet.)

BOOKS LIZZIE HAS RECENTLY ENJOYED HAVING READ TO HER:

Marlee and Ben Alex, *Grandpa and Me*, Lion Publishing.

Roald Dahl, *The BFG*, Puffin.

Roald Dahl, *Charlie and the Chocolate Factory*, Puffin.

C.S.Lewis, *The Chronicles of Narnia*, Collins. (Also available on cassette.)

Little Lion Bible Stories, Lion Publishing and *Palm Tree Bible Stories*, Palm Tree Press: two series of inexpensive, well-illustrated modern versions of Bible stories.

Anne Rooke, *I'm Louise*, Learning Development Aids. (A simple book about a girl with Down's Syndrome, the story as told by her.)

Patricia St John, *Treasures of the Snow* and other books, Scripture Union.

GAMES

The Balloon Game (colour matching).

Connect4 (counting skills and patterns).

Dominoes (Galt produce large, clear colour-coded ones).

Ladybirds (a numbers 1–6 card game).

Learning to Spell, Michael Stanfield.

Lotto games, for example 'Fun Numbers'.

Peephole (matching and remembering parts of pictures; Galt).

Picture Pairs by 'Big Box'.

Sorry (counting and reading instructions).

Sound Tracks and Tongue Twisters (two games from Living and Learning which use listening skills to play a kind of lotto).

SOFTWARE

Computer programmes for the BBC machine, available from Learning Development Aids (Educational Software Dept): *The Best 4*, including *Podd* (ASK Software); *Colour Copter*, *Early Reading*, *Pick a word* (all ESM); *Red Riding Hood*.

CASSETTES

Many stories are available on tape; they are specially good for car journeys. Lizzie's favourites include *Chronicles of Narnia* and *The Times Tables Set to Music*.

12. Other helpful addresses

UK

MENCAP (Royal Society for Mentally Handicapped Children and Adults), MENCAP National Centre, 123 Golden Lane, London EC1Y 0RT   *Tel.* 071 253 9433

Pre-School Playgroups Association, Alford House, Aveline Street, London SE11 5DJ

Toy Libraries Association, Seabrook House, Wyllyotts Manor, Darkes Lane, Potters Bar, Herts EN6 2HL

British Institute of Mental Handicap, Wolverhampton Road, Kidderminster, Worcestershire DY10 3PP

Revised MAKATON Vocabulary, published by (Mrs Margaret Walker, Project co-ordinator) Makaton Vocabulary Development Project, 85 Pierrefondes Avenue, Farnborough, Hants.
   Makaton is a sign language that has been found to encourage the development of language in Down's children.

EIRE

Down's Syndrome Association of Munster, Moores Fort, Tipperary

USA

Betty A. Green, Down's Syndrome Congress of California, 5832 Scotwood Drive, Rancho Palos Verdes, California 90274

AUSTRALIA

Down's Syndrome Association, PO Box 1556, Brisbane 4001

Association for Developmentally Young Children, PO Box 379, North Quay, Queensland 4000

Mental Health Centre, Perth, Western Australia

Queensland Subnormal Children's Welfare Association, 38 Jordan Terrace, Bowen Hills, Brisbane

Subnormal Children's Welfare Association, 8 Junction Street, Ryde, NSW 2112

Mrs Iris Hallam, Co-ordinator for Down's Syndrome, Darwin Hospital, Casuarina, Darwin, Northern Territory

NEW ZEALAND

New Zealand Society for the Intellectually Handicapped, 6th Floor, Brandon House, Featherston Street, Wellington

SOUTH AFRICA

Mr M. Botha, 14 Windsor Road, Oostersee, Parow 7500

ITALY

Mr Enzo Razzano, Associazione Bambini Down, Presso Razzano, Largo Boccea 33, Rome

MEXICO

Mr J. Alejandro Gonzalez, Retorno 9 No. 5, Col. Avenue, Mexico 21 D.F.

13. Bibliography

V. Axline, *Dibs in Search of Self*, Penguin Books, 1964

Carol Baker, *Reading Through Play*, Macdonald, 1981

S. Buckley, *Teaching Speech Through Reading*, Portsmouth Down's Syndrome Project, 1986

J. Carr, *Young Children with Down's Syndrome*, Butterworth, 1975

C. Cunningham and H. Davis, *Working with Parents: Frameworks for Collaboration*, Oxford University Press

Cliff Cunningham and Patricia Sloper, *Helping your Handicapped Baby*, Souvenir Press, Human Horizons series, 1979

H. Davis and R. Rushton, *Counselling and Supporting Parents of Children with Developmental Delay: A Research Evaluation*, Journal of Mental Deficiency Research, 1989

H. Davis and L. Fallowfield (editors), *Counselling in Health Care,* John Wiley and Sons, 1991

Bill Gillham, *First Sentences* (workbooks and cards available from Learning Development Aids), 1979

Bill Gillham, *First Words Language Programme,* Allen and Unwin, 1979

Bill Gillham, *First Words Picture Book,* Methuen (series of useful books)

Joan Hebden, *She'll Never Do Anything, Dear,* Souvenir Press, 1985

Help Your Child Learn Number Skills, Usborne Parents' Guides, 1989

Jan Lloyd, *Jacob's Ladder,* Picador, 1984

Hazel Morgan, *Through Peter's Eyes,* Arthur James—the story of a Down's boy who cannot speak: life through his eyes, written by his mother, 1990

Henri Neuwen, *The Road to Daybreak,* Darton, Longman and Todd, 1985

Carolyn Nystrom, *The Trouble with Josh,* Lion Publishing: a book on mental handicap in the Lion Care series for children, 1989

Brenda Pettenuzza, *I Have Down's Syndrome,* Franklin Watts, 1987

Portage Manual, NFER—Nelson Publications

Portage: Progress, Problems and Possibilities, NFER—Nelson Publications, 1988

Portage: More than a Teaching Programme? NFER—Nelson Publications, 1986

Portage: Pre-schoolers, Parents and Professionals, NFER—Nelson Publications, 1986

Portage: The Importance of Parents, NFER—Nelson Publications, 1985

Extending and Developing Portage, NFER—Nelson Publications, 1987

Libby Purves, *How Not to Be a Perfect Mum,* Fontana

Jean Vanier, *The Broken Body,* Darton, Longman and Todd

Westmacott and Cameron, *Behaviour Can Change,* Macmillan, 1981

M. White and K. East, *The Wessex Revised Portage Language Checklist,* NFER—Nelson Publications, 1983

Other titles from LION PUBLISHING: